Investigations in
DERMATOLOGY

Investigations in
DERMATOLOGY

Editors

Sanjeev Gupta MD DNB
Professor and Head
Department of Dermatology
MM Institute of Medical Sciences and Research
Mullana, Ambala, Haryana, India

Rohit Batra MD
Consultant Dermatologist
Sir Ganga Ram Hospital
New Delhi, India

Sumit Gupta MD
Consultant Dermatologist
Sir Ganga Ram Hospital
New Delhi, India

Managing Editor

Saurabh Swaroop Gupta MD DNB
Assistant Professor
Department of Dermatology
MM Institute of Medical Sciences and Research
Mullana, Ambala, Haryana, India

Forewords

Shyam Verma
Archana Singal

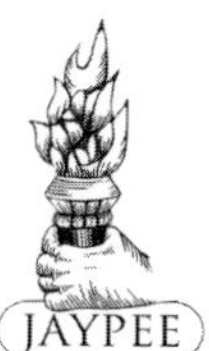

JAYPEE BROTHERS MEDICAL PUBLISHERS
The Health Sciences Publisher
New Delhi | London

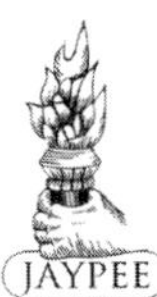 **Jaypee Brothers Medical Publishers (P) Ltd**

Headquarters
EMCA House
23/23-B, Ansari Road, Daryaganj
New Delhi 110 002, India
Landline: +91-11-23272143, +91-11-23272703
+91-11-23282021, +91-11-23245672
E-mail: jaypee@jaypeebrothers.com

Corporate Office
Jaypee Brothers Medical Publishers (P) Ltd.
4838/24, Ansari Road, Daryaganj
New Delhi 110 002, India
Phone: +91-11-43574357
Fax: +91-11-43574314
E-mail: jaypee@jaypeebrothers.com

Overseas Office
JP Medical Ltd.
83, Victoria Street, London
SW1H 0HW (UK)
Phone: +44-20 3170 8910
Fax: +44(0)20 3008 6180
E-mail: info@jpmedpub.com

Website: www.jaypeebrothers.com
Website: www.jaypeedigital.com

Investigations in Dermatology / Sanjeev Gupta, Rohit Batra, Sumit Gupta

First Edition: **2023**

ISBN: 978-93-5465-513-5

Printed at: SDR Printers

Dedicated to

Our Teachers
For nurturing and full-filling our academic aspirations

Our Parents
For their belongings, true affection and unconditional love

Our Wives and Children
Dr Sunita Gupta, Namya and Gauri (Sanjeev Gupta)
Dr Neha Batra, Aarna (Rohit Batra)
Dr Rhythm, Vikramaditya (Sumit Gupta)
For their understanding, forbearance, and unconditional support

Our Patients
For providing us an opportunity to serve them and learn from them

CONTRIBUTORS

EDITORS

Sanjeev Gupta MD DNB
Professor and Head
Department of Dermatology
MM Institute of Medical Sciences and Research
Mullana, Ambala, Haryana, India

Rohit Batra MD
Consultant Dermatologist
Sir Ganga Ram Hospital
New Delhi, India

Sumit Gupta MD
Consultant Dermatologist
Sir Ganga Ram Hospital
New Delhi, India

MANAGING EDITOR

Saurabh Swaroop Gupta MD DNB
Assistant Professor
Department of Dermatology
MM Institute of Medical Sciences and Research
Mullana, Ambala, Haryana, India

CONTRIBUTING AUTHORS

Aastha Sharma MD
Speciality Consultant
Department of Dermatology
University Hospital of North Durham
Durham, United Kingdom

Ajinkya Gujrathi MD
Senior Resident
MM Medical College and Hospital
Solan, Himachal Pradesh, India

Akriti Gakhar MD
Consultant Dermatologist
New Delhi, India

Amit Mittal MD
Professor and Head
Department of Radiodiagnosis
MM Institute of Medical Sciences and Research
Mullana, Ambala, Haryana, India

Amit Soni MD DM
Associate Professor
Department of Gastroenterology
Shri Guru Ram Rai Institute of Medical and Health Sciences
Dehradun, Uttarakhand, India

Aneet Mahendra MD
Professor, Department of Dermatology, MM Institute of Medical Sciences and Research, Mullana, Ambala, Haryana, India

Anuradha Yadav MD
Senior Resident
Department of Dermatology
MM Institute of Medical
Sciences and Research
Mullana, Ambala, Haryana,
India

Arushi Gakhar MD
Consultant Dermatologist
New Delhi, India

Deeksha Goyal MD
Senior Resident
Department of Dermatology
MM Institute of Medical
Sciences and Research
Mullana, Ambala, India

Himanshu Singla MD
Consultant Radiologist
Singla Clinic and
Ultrasound Centre
Ambala, Haryana, India

Jasleen Kaur
Department of Dermatology
MM Institute of Medical
Sciences and Research
Mullana, Ambala, Haryana,
India

Meghna Khatri
Department of Dermatology
MM Institute of Medical
Sciences and Research
Mullana, Ambala, Haryana,
India

Namya Gupta
Kalpana Chawla Government
Medical College
Karnal, Haryana, India

Narender Kaur MD
Professor and Head
Department of Microbiology
MM Institute of Medical
Sciences and Research
Mullana, Ambala, Haryana,
India

Nidhi Jindal MD
Consultant Dermatologist
Apollo Clinic and Oliva Skin
and Hair Clinic
Kolkata, West Bengal, India

Pradhuman DNB
Senior Resident
Department of Radiology
SGT Medical College Hospital
and Research Institute
Gurugram, Haryana, India

Rachita Dhurat MD
Professor and Head
LTM Medical College
Sion, Mumbai, Maharashtra,
India

Rohit Batra MD
Consultant Dermatologist
Sir Ganga Ram Hospital
New Delhi, India

Rohit Singla MD
Associate Professor
Department of Dermatology
MM Institute of Medical
Sciences and Research
Mullana, Ambala, Haryana,
India

Sanjeev Gupta MD DNB
Professor and Head
Department of Dermatology
MM Institute of Medical
Sciences and Research
Mullana, Ambala, Haryana,
India

Saurabh Swaroop Gupta
MD DNB
Assistant Professor
Department of Dermatology
MM Institute of Medical
Sciences and Research
Mullana, Ambala, Haryana,
India

Sumeet Pethe MD
Consultant Dermatologist
Suresh Vasant Pethe Skin
Clinic
Pune, Maharashtra, India

Sumit Gupta MD
Consultant Dermatologist
Sir Ganga Ram Hospital
New Delhi, India

Sunita Gupta MD
Professor and Head
Department of General
Medicine
MM Institute of Medical
Sciences and Research
Mullana, Ambala, Haryana,
India

Udya Chauhan
Department of Dermatology
MM Institute of Medical
Sciences and Research
Mullana, Ambala, Haryana,
India

Vivek Singh
Department of Dermatology
MM Institute of Medical
Sciences and Research
Mullana, Ambala, Haryana,
India

FOREWORD

It is a pleasure to write this foreword for this novel book edited by three young, dynamic, well-informed dermatologists who also happen to be good friends who I have known for several years. It is indeed a bright thought to conceive the idea of such a book that deals with an aspect which is "so close and yet so far" for practicing dermatologists. Bob Dylan's famous song "The Times They Are A-Changin" rings so true here! Gone are the days when dermatology was a purely visually oriented field, practiced in a small, well-lit room with good lighting and a magnifying lens being its most important prerequisites. Advances and modernization of dermatology are invariably accompanied by the need as well as the urge 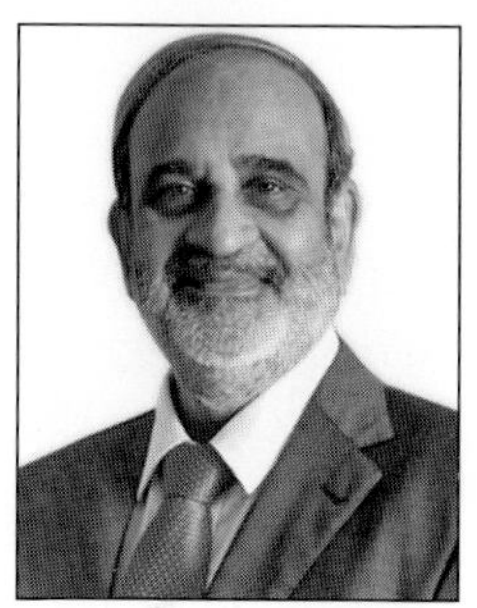 to order more investigations for accuracy and documentation. Some investigations, however, are ordered or performed mechanically and out of habit. A busy practitioner juggling his time between clinical examination and procedures often does not find time to read indications and relevance for several investigations. This handy book, edited by an astute clinician–academician and two well-trained seasoned dermatologists, will meet that need of a ready reference for the busy practitioner. Authors chosen by them are hand-picked and there is no doubt that they will do justice to their topics. I congratulate the editors and the authors for conceiving and executing the writing of this ready reckoner. I truly hope that it is widely circulated and read.

Shyam Verma MBBS DVD PhD FRCP (London)
Consultant Dermatologist, Vadodara, India
Founding Editor of Indian Dermatology Online Journal
International Board Member of European Academy of Dermatology and Venereology
Vice President of International Society of Dermatology

FOREWORD

I feel privileged to write the foreword for the 1st edition of *Investigations in Dermatology*, edited by Drs Sanjeev Gupta, Rohit Batra, and Sumit Gupta. This book obviously fills the existing gap in the management of dermatologic patients.

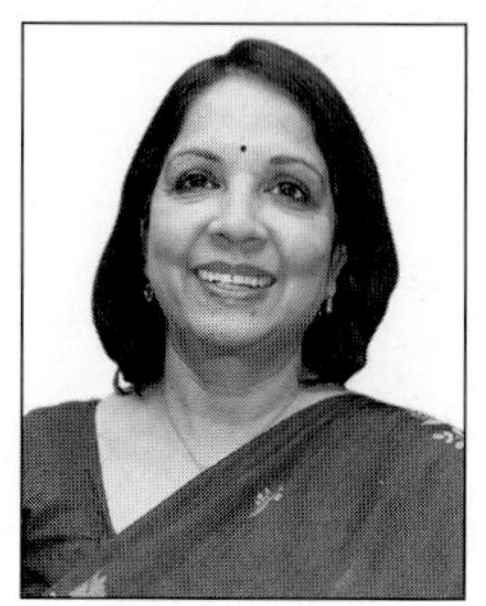

Dermatology, earlier considered to be an allied medical specialty to medicine, is a very fast evolving discipline. Presence of skin lesions carries a huge psychosocial burden and should be addressed effectively and accurately. Skin lesions are amenable to visual examination, and their morphology, configuration, site of lesions, and age of onset often give a clue to varied differential diagnoses. Likewise, skin lesions are also most prone to self-medication, especially in a country where most drugs (topical or systemic) are available over the counter without prescription with resultant change in morphology and difficulty in arriving at a correct diagnosis. Thus, the final diagnosis is reached at after conducting various office or laboratory investigations. In addition, majority of skin diseases are not limited to the skin and have a systemic component or association, whose presence and extent need exploration. This fact is coupled with fast-expanding therapeutic armamentarium including immunosuppressives, biologics/biosimilar, etc., which require pretreatment/baseline and periodic laboratory monitoring.

Akin to therapeutics, diagnostic modalities are evolving very fast; some are simple and can be carried out in the office with immediate results while for others some hours to days are required. Knowledge of these laboratory tests, their right indications, and interpretation requires sound knowledge of the disease process. This book is an excellent attempt to offer comprehensive description of the rationale, procedure, and interpretation of dermatologic diseases–related office procedures and hematological, histological (including specialized tests such as direct and indirect immunofluorescence), and radiological investigations, required for the management of skin diseases. Generous use of diagrammatic representations, flowchart, and tables is a unique reader-friendly feature. This book fills an obvious gap in the management of skin diseases and seems to be a must-have book for each and every practitioner.

I congratulate all the editors for their brilliant concept and flawless execution and wish them best of luck in their academic endeavor.

Archana Singal MD FAMS
Director Professor and Head, Dermatology and STD
University College of Medical Sciences and
GTB Hospital, New Delhi, India
Associate Section Editor, British Journal of Dermatology
Editor Elect-IJDVL (2022)
Founding President Nail Society of India (NSI) 2012–2020

PREFACE

विद्या ददाति विनयं विनयाद् याति पात्रताम्।
पात्रत्वाद् धनमाप्रोति धनाद्धर्मं ततः सुखम्।।

"Knowledge makes one humble, humility begets worthiness, worthiness creates wealth and enrichment, enrichment leads to right conduct, right conduct brings contentment."

Skin diseases are considered to be the mirror image of internal diseases. Although most of the skin diseases are usually diagnosed by simple visual inspection, yet laboratory investigations are required in several clinical circumstances. Various systemic and internal disorders manifest in the skin directly and indirectly; therefore, we require a number of investigations to rule out or confirm the diagnosis. Investigations in dermatology may be necessary to make a diagnosis or to reassure the patient that there is nothing more sinister underlying their skin manifestation. Because of advancement in understanding of etiopathogenesis of various diseases of dermatology and internal medicine and introduction of biologics, the need of various investigations has tremendously increased in the recent past. It is the moral and ethical duty of treating doctors to have better understanding and knowledge of basic interpretation of all the investigations, rather than referring to other specialties.

After so many years in the field, we realized that there was a sparsity of one dedicated book which covered all the investigations required in clinical practice. So, we tried to accept this challenge and are hence presenting you our book on investigations. Welcome to our book *"Investigations in Dermatology"*. This book will throw light and enlighten the readers with interpretation, usefulness, and limitation of all diagnostic procedures used in dermatology and internal medicine.

The book is illustrative with multiple figures and flowcharts and also includes salient features and summary at the end of each chapter. It will not only be of practical importance for dermatologists but will also provide great benefit to all undergraduate and postgraduate students, internists, and family practitioners practicing in India as well as worldwide.

We thank all contributors for finishing this herculean task in time. It has been a pleasure and vast learning experience with an excellent team of authors and editorial board members. We would also like to thank our patients and students who directly and indirectly motivated us to accept this challenge. We will be failing in our duty if we do not thank our family who supported, motivated, and tolerated us for stealing their precious family time.

Special thanks to publisher Shri Jitendar P Vij (Group Chairman), Mr Ankit Vij (Managing Director), Mr MS Mani (Group President), Dr Richa Saxena (Associate Director—Professional Publishing), Ms Pooja Bhandari (Production Head), Ms Upasana Kak (Development Editor), and all members of M/s Jaypee Brothers Medical Publishers (P) Ltd, New Delhi, India, for invaluable contribution.

Happy reading!

Sanjeev Gupta
Rohit Batra
Sumit Gupta

CONTENTS

Cyto-histopathological Examination, Wood's Lamp and Patch Test

Chapter 1A: Cyto-histopathological Investigations in Dermatology

Sanjeev Gupta, Arushi Gakhar, Sumit Gupta, Sumeet Pethe, Rohit Batra,
Ajinkya Gujrathi, Anuradha Yadav

INTRODUCTION

In any disease, laboratory investigations supplement case history and clinical examination in gathering more information for reaching a diagnosis. The common investigations related to dermatological diseases include—Blood investigations, microscopic examinations (bed side tests, and tests done by Microbiology/Pathology department). The related investigations to these are discussed below.

MICROSCOPY

Sanjeev Gupta, Arushi Gakhar

Three well-known techniques of microscopy are: Electron, optical, and scanning probe microscopy.

Optical microscopy is of four types:
1. Dark field
2. Bright field
3. Phase contrast
4. Fluorescence

DARK GROUND MICROSCOPY

It is a technique to visualize unstained samples. In this technique the objects appear bright against dark background. Here, a special condenser is used which has a central obstruction with outer illuminating ring. Some part of light enters the sample and some is scattered, the part of light which is deflected upward into the objective lens helps in visualization and thus the rest of the portion appears dark.

Dark field microscope still remains one of the simplest and most reliable method for the direct detection of *Treponema pallidum*. A small drop of the serous exudate from the lesion is taken on a coverslip. This coverslip is then placed upside down on a clean glass slide. A drop of oil is placed on the condenser. Dark field microscopy removes the unscattered light from the diffraction pattern formed at the rear focal plane of objective which is an advantage over brightfield microscopy resulting in high contrast images (**Table 1**). Objects in dark ground

TABLE 1: Differences between bright field and dark field microscopy.	
Bright field	**Dark field**
Normal wide-field illumination method	An opaque disk is placed underneath condenser lens
Bright background	Dark background
Low contrast	High contrast (structural details)

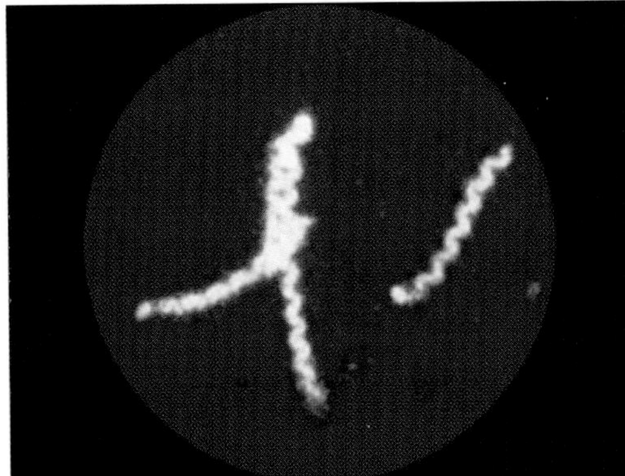

FIG. 1: *Treponema pallidum* in dark ground microscopy.

illumination (DGI) appear remarkably illuminated especially along the edges, outlines, or boundaries. Even the objects with low contrast show brilliant illumination, making for a spectacular sight. Spirochetes like *Treponema pallidum* exhibit illuminated spiral structure and characteristic movement like to and fro movement, corkscrew movement, or bending movement (**Fig. 1**).

ELECTRON MICROSCOPY

- An electron microscope is a microscope that uses a beam of accelerated electrons as a source of illumination.
- It is a special type of microscope providing a high resolution of images, able to magnify even nanometric objects. Images are formed by controlled use of electrons in vacuum, captured on a phosphorescent screen.

- *Fixation*: Most commonly used fixatives are osmium tetroxide, glutaraldehyde, and paraformaldehyde.
- *Dehydration*: By using acetone or ascending concentration of alcohol for a duration of 5–15 minutes.
- *Clearing agent*: Propylene oxide.

Electron microscope is a sophisticated investigation, not required routinely. It is indicated where routine histopathology and immunohistochemistry (IHC) are not able to reveal any conclusive diagnosis. It is useful in:

- Ultrastructural study of Cells and their organelles.
- Some epithelial tumors (identification of intercellular junctions)
- Melanocytic tumors, etc. (identification of melanosomes)
- It is also useful in detailed study of cases of epidermolysis bullosa (subtype determination), Fabry's disease, and amyloidosis.

Electron microscopy is not preferred on prestored and preformed paraffin-embedded blocks.

Disadvantages:
- Electron microscopy (EM) is not economical—it requires stable high voltage supply, vacuum system, etc.
- Findings unlikely to influence treatment, IHC and light microscopy (LM) together are confirmatory in most cases.
- Specimen preparation is tough.
- Only a small proportion of neoplasms can be studied.
- Misinterpretation of non-neoplastic elements of the tumor.
- Availability is a big issue.

Mounting

The "mount" is the way in which a specimen is placed on the slide.

There are three types of mounting:
1. *Wet mount*: The specimen is suspended in a liquid medium between the slide

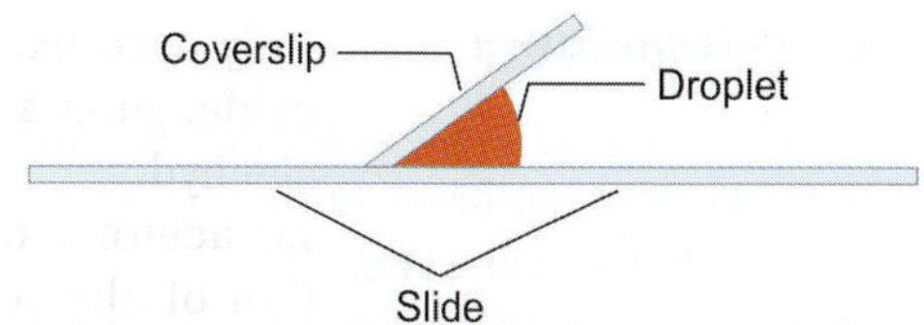

FIG. 2: Wet mount preparation.

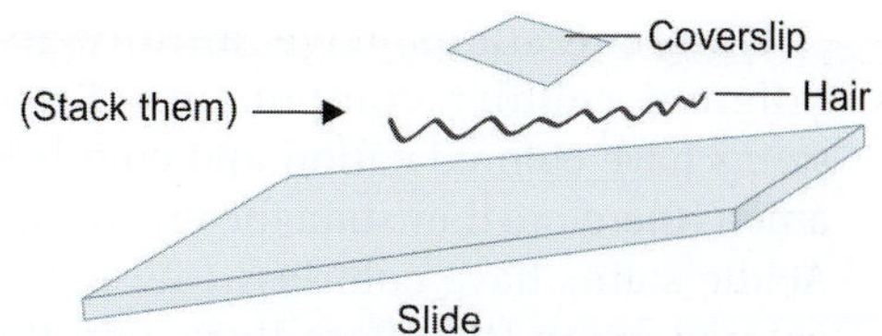

FIG. 4: Dry mount preparation.

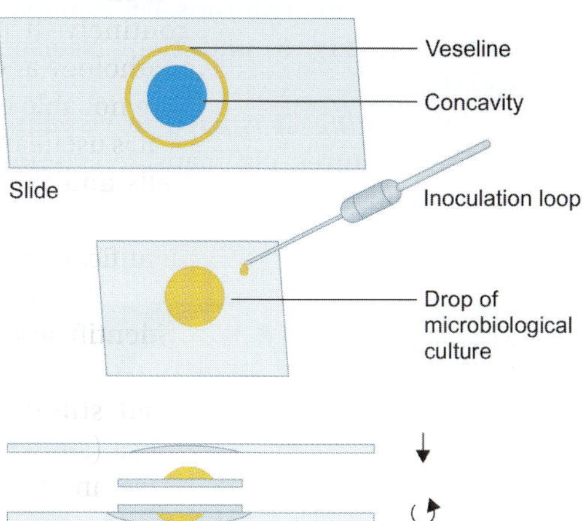

FIG. 3: Steps for hanging drop preparation.

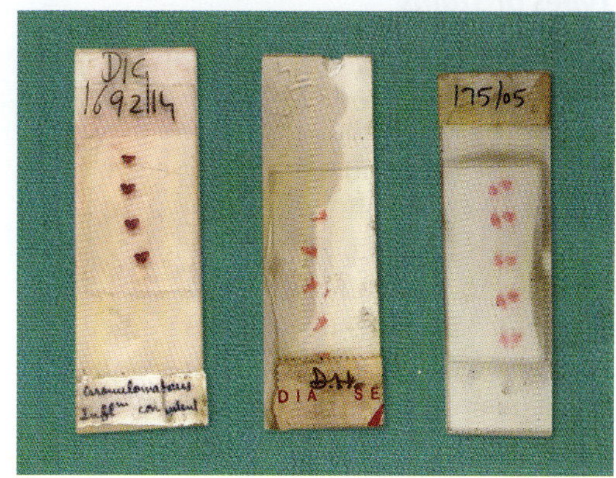

FIG. 5: Slides showing prepared mount.

and coverslip, e.g., potassium hydroxide (KOH) mount (**Fig. 2**).

Hanging drop preparation is a special type of wet mount often used to observe the motility of bacteria. In this method, a drop of bacterial culture is placed on a coverslip which is encircled with petroleum jelly or any other sticky material. The coverslip and drop are then inverted over the well of a depression slide. The drop hangs from the coverslip, and the petroleum jelly forms a seal that prevents evaporation (**Fig. 3**). This preparation gives good view of microbial motility.

2. *Dry mount*: It is the simplest kind of mounting, in which specimen is merely placed on the slide. A coverslip may be placed on top, e.g., hair (**Fig. 4**).

3. *Prepared mount*: The specimens need to be thinly sliced which is usually done with the help of a microtome. The specimen is then dehydrated and stained. In order to protect the specimen from decay, a fixative is used. For example, hematoxylin and eosin (H&E) stain (**Fig. 5**).

Staining

Stains are organic compounds used to differentiate color either the dead or living organisms against the background for better visualization. It is essentially a dye made up of two components (groups).

1. *Auxochrome*: Binds to the organism, responsible for acidic or basic nature of the dye. Basic dyes are positively charged which bind to the bacterial cells surface as it contains acidic polysaccharides and nucleic acids responsible for the opposite (negative) charge. Similarly acidic dyes are negatively charged so they bind to the positively charged cellular components like proteins.

2. *Chromophore*: Forms the colored portion of the stain.

Different stains have affinity for different cellular components. Basic stains have colored cation and colorless anion (therefore they stain the organism). Acidic stains have colorless cation and colored anion (therefore they stain the background).

Types of Stains

- *Basic*: Contains positively charged ions which combine with negatively-charged particles and cellular components such as nucleic acid and acidic polysaccharides. For example, hematoxylin, methylene blue, safranine, crystal violet, basic fuchsin, malachite green, etc.
- *Acidic*: Contains negatively charged ions which combine with positively-charged cellular components. For example, eosin, Indian ink, acid fuchsin, and rose Bengal.
- *Neutral*: Contains both positively and negatively charged ions, imparts different colors to different components, e.g., Giemsa's stain.

  Giemsa stain is a buffered thiazine-eosinate solution used to differentiate nuclear and/or cytoplasmic morphology of platelets, red blood cells (RBCs), white blood cells (WBCs), bacteria and parasites (**Fig. 6**).

Staining Techniques

- *Simple staining*: Single stain is used in this, imparts same color to all the organisms, e.g., methylene blue (**Fig. 7**).
- *Differential staining*: In this technique, two different stains are used along with a decolorizing agent which gives different color to different organisms. For example, Gram stain (**Fig. 8**) and Ziehl–Neelsen (ZN) stain.
- *Special staining*: It is used to visualize special structures, e.g., capsule staining (**Fig. 9**, **Table 2**).

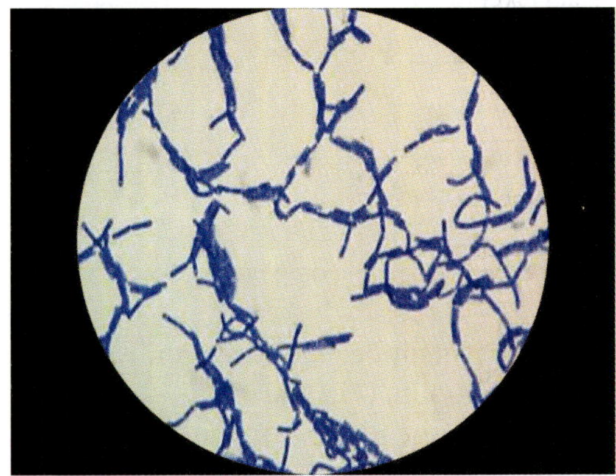

FIG. 7: Simple staining with methylene blue.

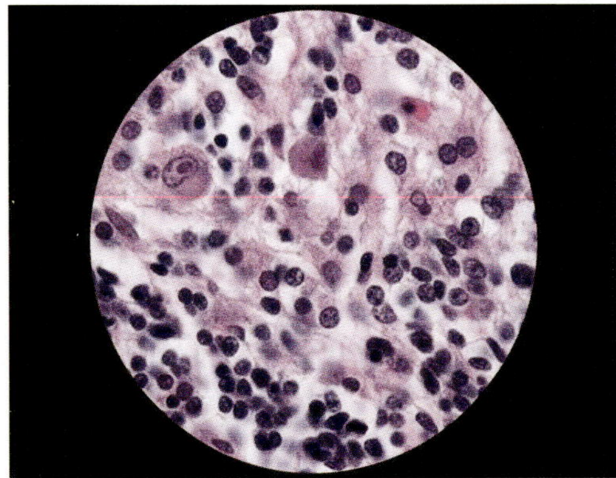

FIG. 6: Giemsa stain (neutral stain).

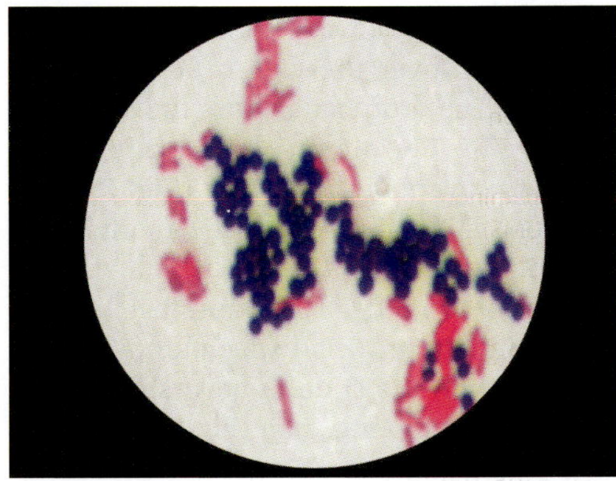

FIG. 8: Differential staining by Gram stain.

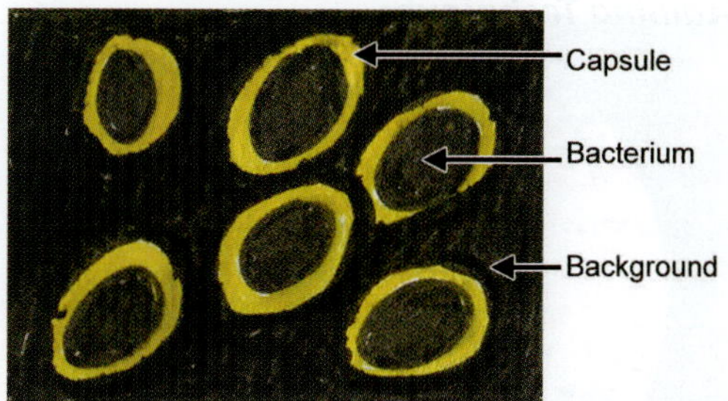

FIG. 9: Special staining of the capsule of the bacteria.

TABLE 2: Special stains used in dermatology.

Special stains	Tissue constituent	Color
Periodic acid–Schiff (PAS)	Glycogen and mucopolysaccharide	Magenta red
Congo red	Amyloid	Red with green birefringence
Masson trichrome	Collagen and muscle	Green and red, respectively
Perl's Prussian blue	Iron	Blue
Von Kossa	Calcium	Brown/black
Alizarin Red	Calcium	Red
Sudan Black	Fat	Black
Oil Red O	Fat	Red
Masson's Fontana	Melanin	Black
Alcian blue	Acid mucopolysaccharide	Blue
Toluidine blue	Mast cells	Metachromatic purple
Van Gieson	Collagen	Red
Grocott's methenamine silver (GMS) staining	Fungi	• Fungi and melanin—black • Mucin and glycogen—dark gray

Uses of fixation:
- It kills bacteria making handling of the specimen safer.

- It prevents autolysis by inactivating the autolytic enzymes.
- It increases the permeability of cells to stain.
- It unfolds the globular proteins and exposing reactive groups and increasing affinity for stain.

HEMATOXYLIN AND EOSIN STAIN

This is the most common stain used for staining most of the biopsy specimen. Hematoxylin is a dye which is extracted from a logwood tree (found in Central America and Mexico). Eosin is derived from fluorescein which is a synthetic dye. Hematoxylin gives blue color and eosin imparts pink color to the cytoplasm and connective tissue (protein) in the specimen (**Fig. 10**).

Steps of H&E staining:
- Deparaffinization (removal of paraffin wax using xylene)
- Hydration (graded alcohols to water)
- Nuclear staining—using hematoxylin
- Differentiation—acid alcohol
- Bluing—ammonia water
- Counterstaining—using eosin
- Dehydration (application of graded alcohol to 100% alcohol)

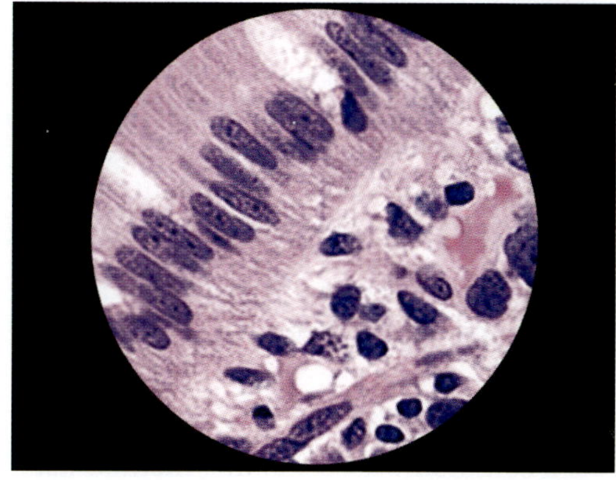

FIG. 10: Hematoxylin and eosin staining.

- Clearing—xylene (transition from alcohol to nonaqueous reagents)

Spore Staining

When vegetative cells of certain bacteria such as *Clostridium perfringens, C. botulinum, C. tetani, Bacillus anthracis,* and *Bacillus cereus* are subjected to environmental stress, they produce dormant forms called endospores. Spore formation (sporulation) occurs when nutrients, such as sources of carbon and nitrogen are depleted, they help in the survival of the organisms during adverse environmental conditions. They do not have a role in reproduction. Endospores are more resistant to heat, dehydration, radiation, and chemicals.

Procedure:
- Prepare a smear, air dry, and heat fix the specimen
- Place the slide over a beaker of boiling water
- Place a small piece of blotting paper over the smear
- Flood the smear with malachite green and leave for 5 minutes
- Remove the blotting paper, let it cool down, and then wash with water
- Counterstain with safranine for 1 minute
- Wash with water, air dry and examine under oil immersion lens.

Primary stain (malachite green) is used to stain the endospores. Because endospores resist staining, the malachite green will be forced into the endospores by heating. In this technique, heating acts as a mordant. Water is used to decolorize the vegetative cells.

Result: Vegetative bacilli appear pink/red while spores appear green.

Gram's Staining

It is a commonly used staining method used to segregate or differentiate organisms based

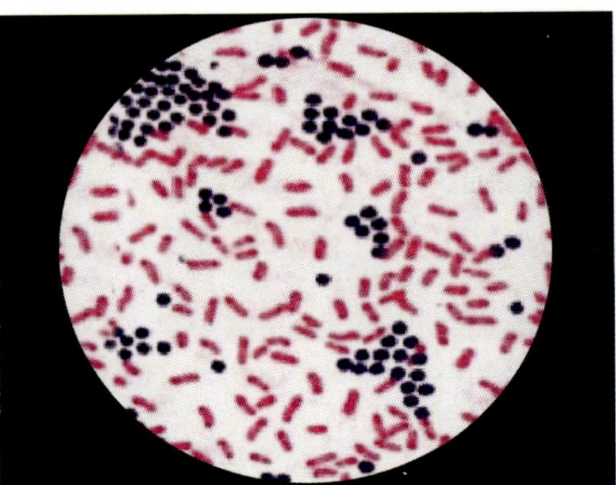

FIG. 11: Gram stain showing gram positive cocci and gram negative bacilli.

on the physical properties and chemical nature of their cell wall into two groups, i.e., gram positive and negative.

Gram positive organism: Cell wall is composed of peptidoglycan mostly with teichoic acid cross linkages which provides resistance against decolorization.

Gram negative organism: Cell wall is composed of large amount of lipids with negligible amount of peptidoglycan, therefore gets decolorized easily.

As a general rule, all cocci are gram positive, except gonococci. And all bacilli are gram negative, except *Bacillus, Clostridium,* and *Corynebacterium* (**Fig. 11**).

Reagents used are:
- *Primary stain*: Gentian violet
- *Mordant:* Gram's iodine
- *Decolorizer*: Acetone/alcohol
- *Counterstain*: Safranine (**Table 3**)

Procedure:
- Spread a thin layer of specimen on a glass slide, dry, and heat fix the specimen.
- Cover the smear with gentian violet for 1 minute and gently rinse off with water
- Gram's iodine for 1 minute and gently rinse with water

TABLE 3: Steps, reagents and color changes in Gram stain.			
		Cell color	
Stain	**Reagent**	**Gram positive**	**Gram negative**
Primary stain	Gentian violet	Violet	Violet
Mordant	Gram's iodine	Purple	Purple
Decolorizer	Acetone/alcohol	Purple	Colorless
Counterstain	Safranine	Purple	Pink

Shape: Cocci are spherical and bacilli are rod shaped.

- Decolorize by pouring alcohol/acetone over the smear till the blue dye no longer runs off the slide with the decolorizer and wash immediately with water
- Counterstaining with safranine for 1 minute and wash with water
- Air dry and examine under oil immersion

Arrangement: Staphylococci are cocci in clusters and streptococci are cocci in chains. Mycobacterium cannot be stained by Gram's stain because of their high lipid content. Hence, they are being stained by a differential staining technique known as ZN staining.

ZIEHL–NEELSEN STAINING

It is a special stain to differentiate acid fast and non-acid fast micro organisms. For the Dermatologist, there are two main Mycobacteria of clinical importance for which this stain is used in suspected cases— *M. tuberculosis* and *M. leprae*. There is a thick cell wall in mycobacteria composed of mycolic acid which resists the process of decolorization by alcohol and acid as a result of which the property of acid-fastness is attained (**Fig. 12**).

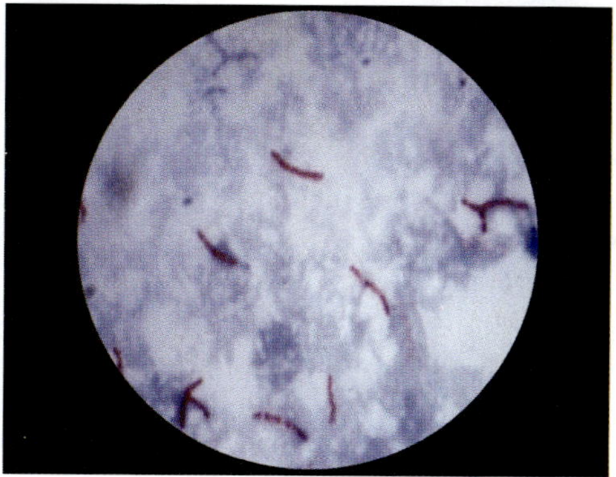

FIG. 12: ZN stain showing acid fast bacilli.

Requirements:
- Glass slide with fixed smear
- Bunsen flame
- Reagents:
  - *Primary stain*: Carbol fuchsin
  - *Decolorizer*: 5% (*M. leprae*) or 20% (*M. tuberculosis*) sulfuric acid/1% HCl in alcohol
  - *Counterstain*: Methylene blue (**Table 4**)

Procedure:
- Prepare a smear on a clear and dry glass slide
- Allow it to dry and fix it with heat, flood smear with carbol fuchsin stain and

TABLE 4: Steps, reagents and color changes in ZN staining.			
		Cell color	
Stain	**Reagent**	**Acid fast**	**Nonacid Fast**
Primary stain	Carbolfuchsin	Red	Red
Decolorizer	Acid alcohol	Red	Colorless
Counterstain	Methylene blue	Red	Blue

heat slide from below till steam rises for 5 minutes. Do not boil the stain.

- Leave it for 5 minutes to cool down
- Wash in running water
- Tilt slide and add decolorizer drop by drop until the red color stops streaming from the smear
- Again, wash with water and counterstain with methylene blue for 30 seconds
- Finally, wash with water, dry it, and examine under oil immersion lens
  - *M. tuberculosis* appear as thin, long acid fast bacilli, while *M. leprae* appear as thick, short, slender bacilli arranged in groups known as globi or 'bundle of cigar' appearance

Bacterial Index (BI) is graded as detailed below:

6+	Over 1,000 bacilli and globi in an average microscopic field
5+	100–1,000 bacilli/average microscopic field
4+	10–100 bacilli/average microscopic field
3+	1–10 bacilli/average microscopic field
2+	1–10 bacilli/10 microscopic fields
1+	1–10 bacilli/100 microscopic fields

Acid-fast bacilli (AFB) characteristics	*Mycobacterium tuberculosis*	*Mycobacterium leprae*
Acid fastness	More acid fast	Less acid fast

Continued

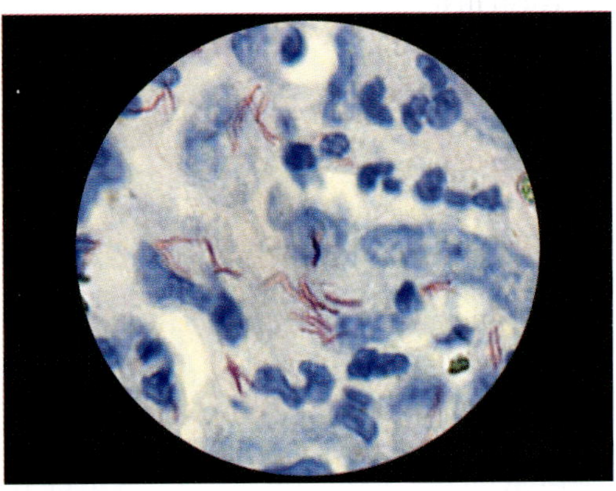

FIG. 13: Acid fast bacilli in ZN stain.

Continued

	Decolorizer	Requires 20% H_2SO_4	Requires 5% H_2SO_4
	Modification	Can be easily stained by ZN technique	Fite-Faraco staining required

Fite-Faraco Stain

It is a modified ZN stain. *M. leprae* is much less acid and alcohol-fast as compared to *Mycobacterium tuberculosis*. The mycolic acid coat of leprosy bacilli is less strong and is easily decolorized by the standard ZN technique. Hence, special stain is used to demonstrate *M. leprae* (**Fig. 13**).

Reagents used are:
- Xylene/peanut oil solution
- Carbol fuchsin solution
- 5% sulfuric acid in 25% alcohol
- Harris hematoxylin/methylene blue

Procedure (Job–Chacko modification):
- Deparaffinize in xylene/peanut oil mixture, two changes, and 6 minutes each
- Drain slides and blot off excess oil
- Wash in running water
- Add carbol fuchsin and leave for 30 minutes
- Wash in tap water
- Decolorize in 5% sulfuric acid in 25% alcohol and two changes of 1.5 minutes each
- Wash in tap water
- Counterstain in Harris hematoxylin for 5 seconds
- Wash in tap water
- Blot and air dry
- Dip in xylene and apply coverslip

Result: Acid-fast bacilli stains red while background stains blue.

POTASSIUM HYDROXIDE SMEAR FOR FUNGAL EXAMINATION

It is used mainly for superficial fungal infections. The superficial fungal infection remain mainly in stratum corneum of epidermal layer but because of thick keratinocyte, the fungal elements are not visualized. KOH preparation causes dissolution of keratinocytes as a result of which fungal elements (hyphae and spores) are properly visualized. The KOH does not allow dissolution of fungal elements.

Sample collection:
Skin: First the site is gently cleaned with spirit to remove any dirt, sebum or topical application. With the help of blunt side of surgical blade, gentle scraping of the scale is done and the sample is collected on the glass slide.

Nails: The distal free end of diseased nail is cut with the help of sterile scalpel blade, scissor, or nail cutter. Along with that, the subungual debris is also collected with any blunt instrument.

Scalp: Diseased hairs are gently plucked with a needle holder or hair plucker. The distal part of the hair is cut, only the proximal 1–2 cm part of hair is kept over slide for examination.

Procedure:
- Place the specimen on a glass slide and cover it with 2–3 drops of 10% KOH solution.
- Apply a coverslip and let the slide sit for 20 minutes for the keratin to dissolve. Press coverslip firmly to obtain monolayer of cells.
- For nail specimen, the clippings should be kept immersed in a KOH solution in a test tube overnight. The slide is then prepared with a drop of this solution as described above. Remove excess KOH using tissue/filter paper.
- Scan the entire preparation at low power (10 × magnification) for fungal elements. Use higher power (40 × magnification) to confirm findings.

Tape method:
- Another method for sample collection uses a piece of transparent cellophane tape applied onto the affected area, firmly pressed and then stripped off in one swift motion, bringing along with it the horny layer of the skin.
- The loaded tape is placed onto the surface of a microscopic glass slide with the sticky surface facing down and pressed into position.
- The tape is gently peeled back at the margins to allow addition of 3–4 drops of 10% KOH and directly visualized under the microscope without a coverslip.
- Advantage of this method is that it is a simpler technique, allows easy

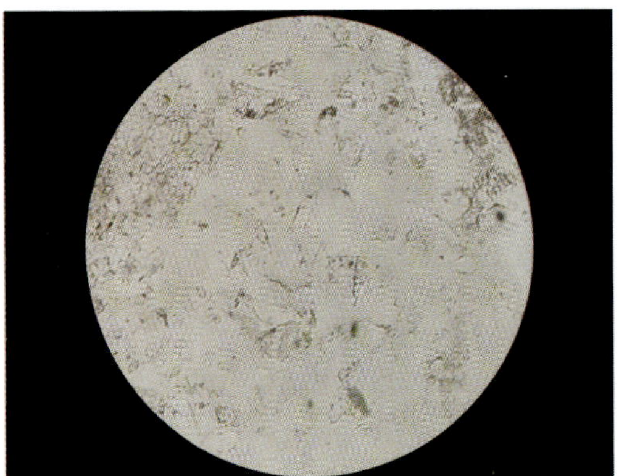

FIG. 14: Fungal hyphae in 10% KOH.

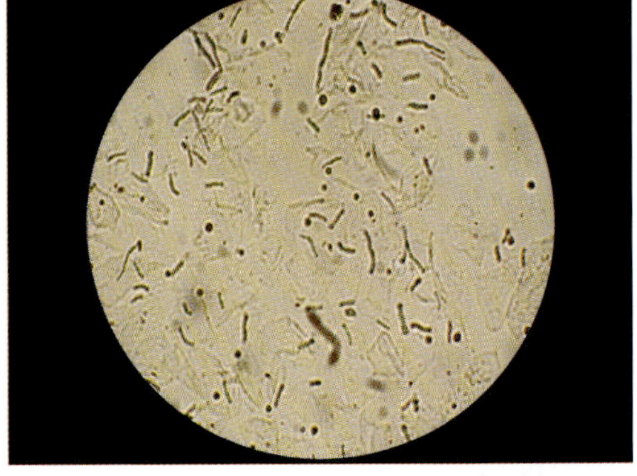

FIG. 15: Pseudohyphae and budding yeast cells in Candidiasis.

transportation and provide a larger area for examination.
- However, the limitation of this technique is it's unsuitability for sample collection in moist areas and for onychomycosis.

Common artefacts:
- Air bubbles
- Oil droplets
- Clothing fibers
- Crystals

These artefacts can give false positive results.

Some common findings in different diseases:
- Dermatophytes—multiple, branched, and septate hyphae (**Fig. 14**)
- Tinea versicolor—hyphae with spores, called "spaghetti and meatballs" appearance
- Candidiasis—budding ovoid yeast cells and pseudohyphae (**Fig. 15**)

SCRAPING FOR SCABIES

Scabies scraping can be used to confirm the presence of the scabies mite, which is <0.5 mm and invisible to the naked eye. The specimens are examined for the mite (**Fig. 16**), eggs, and/or fecal material (scybala).

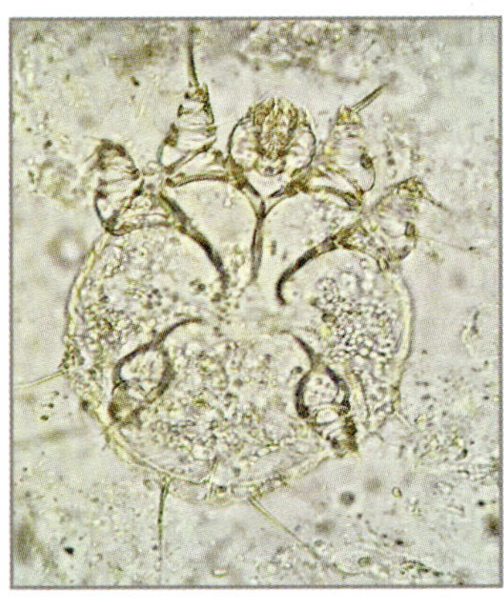

FIG. 16: Sarcoptes scabiei var hominis (Scabies mite).

Procedure:
- Select a burrow or papule (that have not been excoriated) and clean the lesion
- Scrape the burrow or papules with a scalpel blade and smear the contents on a glass slide
- Cover it with 2–3 drops of mineral oil and apply a coverslip. Do not use KOH as this may dissolve the mite's fecal material
- Scan the entire specimen at low power (10 × magnification) for the presence of mites, eggs, and/or fecal material. To confirm the findings use high power (40 × magnification)

TZANCK TEST

Tzanck test is an aid to rapid diagnosis of numerous skin conditions.

Procedure: Select a small, recent, uninfected, intact vesicle and swab with an alcohol pad. If no intact blisters, a crusted lesion or erosion can be used.

- Remove the roof of blister with scissors
- Gently scrape the base of the blister with the blade
- Smear the scrapings on to a glass slide and let it air dry
- Apply 2–3 drops of Giemsa stain (most common), hematoxylin and eosin, methylene blue, papanicolaou or toluidine blue stain
- Leave the stain for 15 minutes
- Then rinse the slide with water and allow it to dry completely
- Examine under oil immersion lens

Acantholytic cells also known as Tzanck cell are seen on Tzanck smear which are rounded cell with round vesicular nucleus, perinuclear halo, peripheral condensation of basophilic cytoplasm and lacks desmosomal connections (**Fig. 17**).

It is used for cytodiagnosis of different disorders like (**Table 5**):

- Pemphigus vulgaris, Pemphigus foliaceus and Hailey–Hailey disease
- Toxic epidermal necrolysis (TEN), Stevens–Johnson syndrome (SJS) and staphylococcal-scalded skin syndrome (SSSS)
- Bullous pemphigoid (BP) and erosive lichen planus
- Basal cell carcinoma
- Herpes simplex, varicella and herpes zoster
- Molluscum contagiosum
- Leishmaniasis

SLIT-SKIN SMEAR EXAMINATION

It is a test in which a sample of material is collected from the skin and then stained for *M. leprae*. It is also used to confirm the diagnosis and classify the disease.

Four routine sites from which sample can be taken:
1. Right earlobe
2. Forehead
3. Chin
4. Left buttock/left upper thigh

Procedure:
- Clean lesion with spirit
- Pinch the fold of skin tightly between your thumb and index finger to drive out blood
- Make an incision in the skin about 5 mm long and 3 mm deep using a size 15 Bard-Parker blade

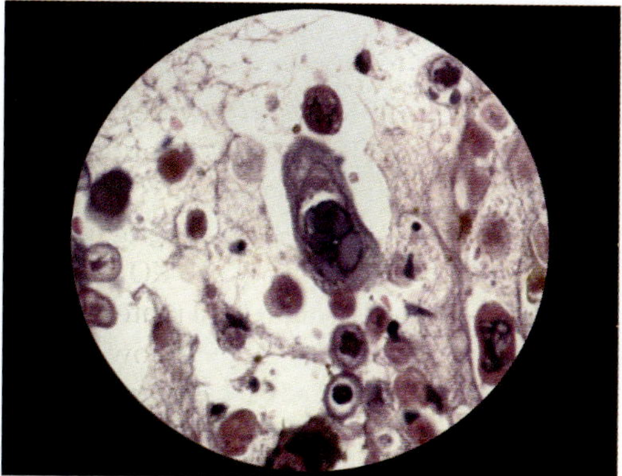

FIG. 17: Tzanck cell in Giemsa stain.

TABLE 5: Tzanck smear findings in bullous disorders.	
Pemphigus	Acantholytic cells
Bullous pemphigoid	Predominantly eosinophils
Chronic bullous disease of childhood	Predominantly neutrophils
Varicella zoster	Multinucleated giant cells
Herpes simplex	Multinucleated giant cells
Toxic epidermal necrolysis	Necrotic cells

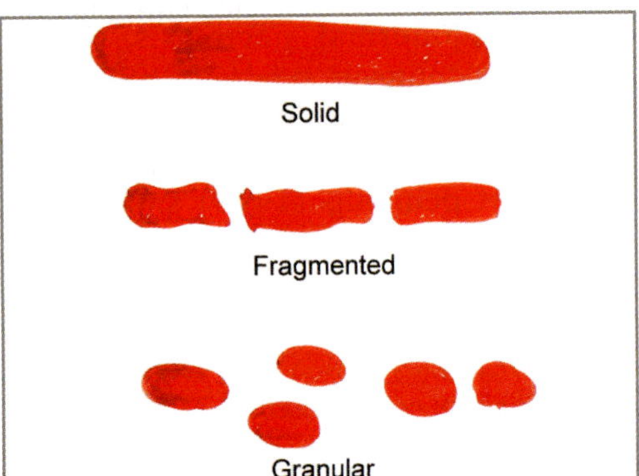

FIG. 18: Diagrammatic representation of different morphology of lepra bacilli in ZN stain.

- Turn the blade at 90° and scrape out fragments of tissue and fluid
- The material obtained is placed on a clean glass slide and made into a smear
- The smear is then dried and heat fixed and then stained by ZN method

Live and viable *M. leprae* are seen as solid stained bacilli, while dead and nonviable are seen as granular, broken or fragmented (**Fig. 18**).

<h2>SKIN BIOPSY</h2>

Sumit Gupta, Sumeet Pethe

SKIN BIOPSY

It is a very common and important outpatient department (OPD) procedure in dermatology practice. A skin biopsy is a procedure in which a sample of skin tissue is removed, processed and examined under a microscope. Special stains can be used to detect bacteria, fungus, immune complexes, lymphocytes, inflammatory mediators etc. Punch biopsy for dermatology use was described by Edward L Keyes in 1887.

Types:
- Punch biopsy
- Shave biopsy
- Incisional biopsy
- Excisional biopsy

Indications of skin biopsy:
- To confirm clinical diagnosis
- As treatment modality in nevi and granuloma annulare
- To evaluate effect of treatment in leprosy where we do biopsy before and after starting treatment

Choice of appropriate time: There are different stages of inflammation in skin as a result of which, type of inflammatory cells keep changing in a lesion overtime, e.g., from neutrophils to lymphocytes to histiocytes. The inflammatory reaction reaches peak level in 24–36 hours from onset of lesion which can be the appropriate time to get the biopsy done. In case of immunofluorescence, the early lesion is preferred because in the late phase immune reactants get consumed.

It is important to collect biopsy from appropriate site (**Table 6**).

Avoid areas that are scratched/excoriated, treated with topical steroids or other

TABLE 6: Biopsy sites of common dermatological disorders.	
Suspected disease	**Biopsy site**
Pemphigus	Small vesicle
Pemphigoid	Avoid large bullae, ulcers, and erosions
Vasculitis	Erythematous/active border of a new lesion
LE	Erythematous/active border of a new lesion
EBA and CBDC	Perilesional/normal skin
Porphyria and pseudoporphyria	Edge of a fresh vesicle (bulla)
Dermatitis herpetiformis	Normally looking perilesional skin 3 mm from a vesicle
Large lesions	The edge, the thickest portion, or the area that is most abnormal in color

(CBDC: chronic bullous disease of childhood; EBA: epidermolysis bullosa acquisita; LE: lupus erythematosus)

anti-inflammatory agents when possible and also important cosmetic areas such as the face and areas with poor healing characteristics (distal lower extremities).

Biopsy of older blisters should be avoided since immune deposits at these sites are degraded and changes such as secondary infection/degeneration can occur.

Preparing the site:
- Clean the area
- Mark the intended lesion with a skin marker
- Langer's lines (exist parallel to the direction of collagen in the dermis) can be demonstrated by gently compressing relaxed skin with the thumb and index finger

Anesthesia: The most commonly used local anesthetic is 1% or 2% lignocaine (lidocaine).

As lidocaine is a vasodilator, small amount of epinephrine is added to constrict the blood vessels, decrease bleeding during the procedure, retards local clearance, hence prolong the anesthesia and reduces risk of systemic toxicity. Avoid the use of epinephrine for acral lesions, tip of nose, or when large quantities are needed, especially in patients with cardiovascular disease.

Contraindication: There are no absolute contraindications for biopsies. However, it should be done with caution in following situations:
- Active infection at the site
- Bleeding diathesis
- Keloidal tendency
- Allergies to local anesthetic

Labeling the specimen is very important and it should include patient and physician name, date of sample collection and location of the lesion from which biopsy was taken.

Punch Biopsy

It is the most easy and economical technique of skin biopsy. The biopsy can be performed with disposable or reusable/autoclavable punches which are available in different sizes ranging from 1 to 10 mm diameter. The biopsy can be for diagnostic or therapeutic purpose.

Procedure:
- Select a punch slightly larger than the lesion.
- Select adequate site and determine the direction of the skin tension lines at the site. Put tension on the skin perpendicular to the observed skin tension lines to create an elliptical wound.
- Place the punch perpendicular to the skin and apply firm and constant downward pressure with a clockwise motion.
- When the punch reaches the subcutaneous fat, there is feeling of give away.
- Remove the punch, elevate the core with forceps and excise it at its base with small tissue scissors or blade.
- Punch biopsies can heal by secondary intention, but punches >3 mm may require closure with suture.
- Clean the wound and apply a dry, nonocclusive dressing.
- Prescribe topical antibiotic for minimum 1 week.

Shave Biopsy

It is removal of representative piece of skin by tangential incision with a blade/scissors.

Indication: Epidermal lesions such as vesiculobullous lesions, seborrheic dermatitis, actinic keratoses, warts, and skin tags.

Advantages:
- Fast
- Good cosmetic result
- Do not require sutures for closure
- It can be used in sensitive anatomic locations where the depth of a punch biopsy puts nerves/blood vessels at risk

Disadvantage: This method is unsuitable for deeper pathologies.

Procedure:
- Stabilize the lesion between the thumb and forefinger.
- A number 15 surgical blade is held parallel to the skin surface and the shave biopsy is performed by using a smooth sweeping stroke rather than a sawing motion.
- Endpoint is pinpoint bleeding which indicates papillary dermis.
- After hemostasis is achieved, ointment and dressing are applied.

It can also be done with:
- Scissors—For pedunculated lesions, it is very easy and effective method.
- Razor blade—In this, we use horizontal sawing motion. It is extremely sharp and hence superficial lesions can be easily removed by this technique.

Incisional Biopsy (Wedge Biopsy)

It is removal of just a small representative part of the lesion for histopathological study.

Indication:
- Lesion larger than 2 cm
- To do special tests such as culture and microscopy
- Dangerous location of the lesion, i.e., near vessels or nerves
- Great suspicion of malignancy

Excisional Biopsy

It is the complete removal of the lesion for microscopic study. As entire lesion is removed, it is both diagnostic and therapeutic.

Advantages:
- Whole specimen is available for histology
- As wound is sutured, it heals with good cosmetic result

Procedure:
- Give suitable local anesthesia
- Align the long axis of the excision parallel to the skin tension lines

- Mark an ellipse around the lesion to be excised, with 30° angles at each apex, the length should be three times the width and a 2- to 5-mm margin of normal skin around the lesion should be included.
- Incise at one apex with a number 15 surgical blade perpendicular to the skin, to cut the tissue with the belly of blade at an angle of 45°.
- Once the ellipse has been incised, lift the sample edge with fine forceps and completely undermine the sample at the level of the subcutaneous fat.

Complications of biopsy: Though rare, the following complications may occur:
- Secondary infection
- Scarring
- Damage to underlying blood vessels or nerves
- Bleeding
- Hematoma formation
- Allergy to adhesive tape
- Allergy to local anesthetic agent (rare)

IMMUNOFLUORESCENCE TEST

Rohit Batra, Ajinkya Gujrathi

IMMUNOFLUORESCENCE TEST

Immunofluorescence (IF) microscopy is a well-established technique that utilizes fluorescent-labeled antibodies to detect specific target antigens in tissues or on cells in suspension. It was pioneered by Coons and Kaplan. It is a gold standard investigation in immunobullous diseases.

Advantages of IF:
- Easy and simple to perform
- Reliable and reproducible
- It is complimentary to biopsy

Principle: There are special dyes which emit fluorescence when exposed to UV-light. This property can be used to detect special proteins (antigen or antibody) when these dyes get conjugated with tissue. Special fluorescent microscope is required for detection of fluorescence. Certain fluorochrome dyes when exposed to UV light emit fluorescent radiation. When these dyes are conjugated to proteins that are subsequently added to tissue sections, the position of the proteins can be traced microscopically by the fluorescence they emit.

Two fluorochromes dyes are generally available:
1. Rhodamine RB200 emits orange fluorescence
2. Fluorescein isothiocyanate emits green fluorescence

Specimen needed:
- Tissue biopsy sample [for direct immunofluorescence (DIF)]
- Serum samples (for indirect IF)

There are four types of tests which are frequently used in dermatology:
1. Direct immunofluorescence
2. Indirect immunofluorescence
3. Complement fixation test
4. Immunoelectron microscopy

DIRECT IMMUNOFLUORESCENCE

Direct immunofluorescence is used to see deposition of different antibodies, e.g., immunoglobulin M (IgM), IgA, IgG, C3, C5b-9 and fibrinogen in skin specimen. It is a single step procedure. The biopsy sample should be kept in liquid nitrogen or in Michel's medium (**Table 7**) (for long distance transportation), if nearby laboratory is available then the sample can be transported in cold normal saline (within 24 hours). After processing of sample in lab, the skin tissue is labeled with fluorescent dye. In case any immune reactants are present in the specimen they emit fluorescence which can be visualized through fluorescent microscope (**Flowchart 1**).

TABLE 7: Transport medium for different studies.	
Type of study	**Transport medium**
Light microscopy H&E	Formalin
Electron microscopy	2.5% glutaraldehyde solution
Immunohisto-chemistry	Formalin fixed paraffin embedded blocks
Direct immunofluorescence	Normal saline, liquid nitrogen, Michel medium, and Zeus medium

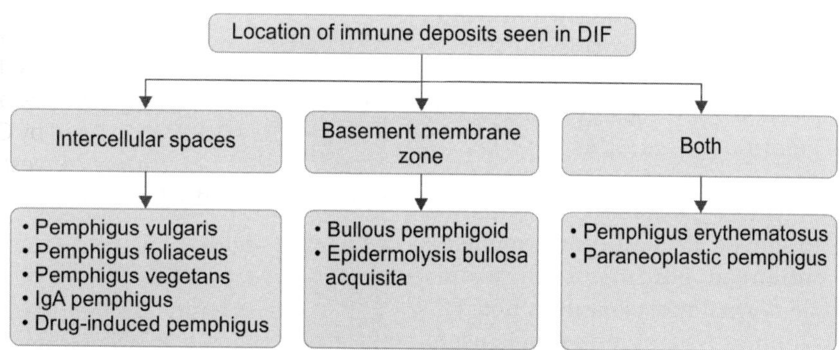

FLOWCHART 1: Sites of immune deposits in various Immunobullous disorders.
(DIF: direct immunofluorescence; IgA: immunoglobulin A)

INDIRECT IMMUNOFLUORESCENCE

Indirect immunofluorescence is a two-step semiquantitative procedure. This is used to detect the autoantibodies in serum or tissue fluids. The choice of substrate is very important for proper results. The main substrates used in frozen sections are monkey esophagus, rat bladder and human salt split skin. The substrate is first incubated with diluted serum for half an hour at room temperature and then washed. Antibodies, if present they get bound to substrate which later on can be detected by incubating with fluorescein isothiocyanate—labeled goat anti-human IgG and/or IgA.

Salt split technique: It is a simple and easy method to distinguish between epidermal and dermal binding autoantibodies.

Method: Incubate the skin sample in 1 M NaCl for 1–2 days at 4°C.

Results:
- Bullous pemphigoid—Roof—antigens will adhere to epidermal side
- Epidermolysis bullosa acquisita (EBA)—Floor—antigens adhere to dermal side

IMMUNOHISTOCHEMISTRY

Immunohistochemistry is the process of detecting proteins in different cells or tissue sections. It also works on the same principle of antigen-antibody binding. The different markers, e.g., radioactive element, fluorescent dye, colloidal gold or enzyme systems, etc., are used in IHC. Since there is no specific antibody to ascertain a specific cell, so a panel of different antibodies is used on formalin fixed, paraffin embedded tissue section in routine practice.

Chapter 1B: Wood's Lamp Examination and Patch Test

Sanjeev Gupta, Anuradha Yadav

Wood's lamps are small, durable, safe, inexpensive and easy to use. These emit ultraviolet (UV) rays, generated by mercury arc fitted with a filter called wood's filter which is made up of nickel oxide and barium silicate. It is opaque to all light rays, except a band between 320 and 400 nm with a peak at 365 nm (**Fig. 19**).

Wood's lamp examination is useful to determine type of melasma, i.e., epidermal, dermal or mixed as epidermal melasma shows enhanced contrast with wood's lamp while dermal melasma does not. This categorization of type of melasma is useful because dermal melasma is less responsive to treatment compared with epidermal melasma (**Table 8**).

Techniques of wood's lamp examination:
- Lamp should be allowed to warm up for around 1 minute

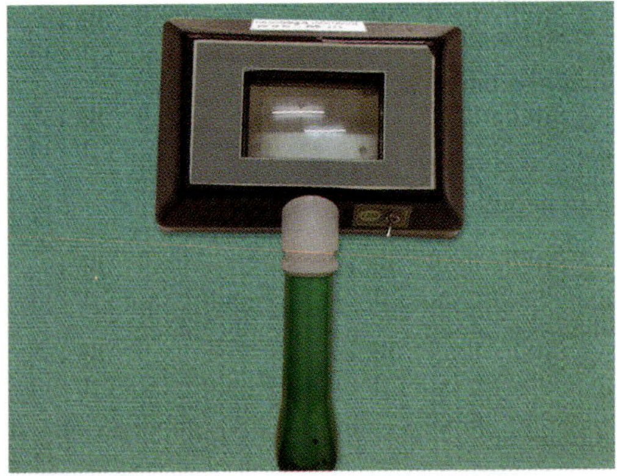

FIG. 19: Wood's lamp

- Examination room should be dark or alternately a black cloth can be used between the visual area of the woods lamp and the lesion.
- Examiner should get dark adapted to see contrast clearly
- Light source should be 4–5 inches from lesion
- Topical medications and soap, etc., should be wiped off from site to be examined since these may fluoresce under wood's light
- Patient's eyes should be covered to prevent injury to retina and conjunctiva

Most common source of error:
- Insufficiently darkened room
- Light reflected from examiner's clothing; white coats/shirts fluoresce because of optical brighteners present in detergents
- Fluorescence produced by ointment

It can also be helpful in diagnosis of premalignant and malignant conditions which involves application of 20% aminolevulinic acid (ALA) ointment to the tumor and leaving it for 4–6 hours under occlusion allowing protoporphyrin IX to accumulate after which it is illuminated with Wood's lamp. Useful for identification of squamous cell epithelioma, basal cell epithelioma, Bowen's disease, etc.

PATCH TEST

Sanjeev Gupta, Anuradha Yadav

PATCH TEST

It is used to identify offending causes/allergens of allergic contact dermatitis.

Procedure:
- Various patch test allergens (contained within small chambers) are held against the patient's back using a paper tape (**Fig. 20**).

TABLE 8: Findings of Wood's lamp examination in common dermatological disorders.	
Disease	**Color with Wood's light**
Vitiligo, ash leaf macules of tuberous sclerosis	White
Melasma (melanin in epidermis), lentigo, freckles, and café au lait spots	Darker than surrounding skin
Tinea capitis due to *Microsporum* species*	Blue-green
Pityriasis versicolor	Yellow
Pityrosporum folliculitis	Blue-white
Acanthosis nigricans	Pink
Erythrasma (caused by *Corynebacterium minutissimum*)	Coral red
Porphyrins in urine, feces, blood, blister fluid, and teeth	Red-pink
Pseudomonas	Green

* Always remember that not all fungus emit fluorescence.

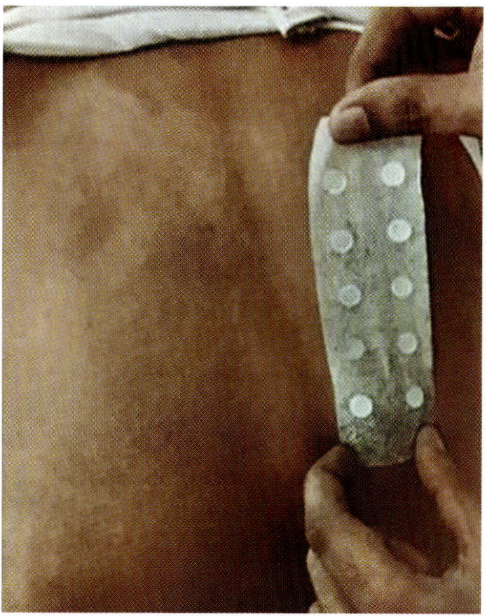

FIG. 20: Method of application of Patch test allergens on patient's back.

- The tape should remain in place for 48 hours during which it should be kept dry
- Read the findings at 48, 72, and 96 hours after application
- The presence of erythema, papules, and/or vesicles indicates a positive test

Principle of Patch Test

Patch testing is based on the fact that activated and antigen specific T-lymphocytes are seen in whole of the body and so the patch tests allergen can be applied to normal skin. When the allergen is applied on normal looking skin area, it produces a definitive dermatitis reaction. The test is a "miniature model" of the disease under investigation. Absorption of the allergen in quantity which is sufficient enough to develop a reproducible inflammation forms the basis of the patch test. A positive patch test gives a confirmation that the individual has allergic contact sensitivity, provided it is applied correctly.

Test material:
1. Allergen
2. Finn chamber on Scanpor tape

Test Procedure

In the test procedure, small quantities of suspected antigens are applied on an area of clinically normal skin (most common site being the upper back) and are occluded with a fixing tape. These are left undisturbed for 48 hours and then removed. The readings are ideally taken 1 hour after patch removal. This delay allows the erythema (caused by striping action of tape on its removal) to settle down. Some allergens, however, may show delayed positivities, e.g., neomycin and corticosteroids, so a second reading should be taken at day 4 and day 7 as well.

Patch Test Units

At present, Finn Chamber, developed by Pirila in 1975, is the most common system used to apply the allergens. It is made of aluminium and has a diameter of 8 mm and a depth of 0.5 mm. An indigenous counterpart of the Finn chamber was used in India by Kaur and Sharma in 1986 where they used the central portions of the metallic caps on the penicillin injection vials. Other chambers are also available like Van der Bend, Epicheck, IQ Ultra and Curatest F.

These chambers are used to ensure occluded contact with skin.

Vehicles

The standard vehicle used is white petrolatum due to its occlusive and hypoallergenic property.

Tapes

The modern tapes have adequate tack and keep the patches in close approximation to the skin surface. The tape used for fixation should ideally be nonocclusive, nonallergenic and nonirritant. If tape peels off, test should be repeated.

Allergens

More than 300 substances are now commercially available as allergens for patch testing. Common allergens used are balsam of Peru, benzocaine, epoxy resin, neomycin, parthenium, potassium dichromate, fragrance mix, etc. The standard series which contains the most common allergens can be supplemented with additional series for the purpose of targeting specific categories of individuals such as hairdressers, housewives, gardeners, dental technicians, printers, etc.

Although any chemical in the environment can act as an allergen causing contact dermatitis, it is recommended that the standard series should be used for patch testing. Using such standardized series, it is possible to detect about 70–80% of the contact sensitivities.

The correct concentration of an allergen will give a moderate reaction in a sensitized person but no reaction in an unsensitized person. For all the standard allergens, the correct patch test concentrations are known. Only the correct amount of the test material should be used for each patch test. Never overfill as it may contaminate the neighboring test sites.

It is best to prepare the allergens on the day of the test and apply immediately to avoid false negative reactions.

Storage of allergens: Allergens are stored in refrigerator at 4°C in dark because many substances are unstable, if exposed to light.

Site:
- Back most commonly used
- Upper arm lateral aspect
- Abdomen
- Thighs

Reading and evaluation of patch test results: Well-established allergens are conventionally tested in such concentrations that a 48 hours exposure under an occlusive patch allows penetration of a sufficient amount to provoke a reaction in a sensitized individual.

The readings should be taken and graded according to the International Contact Dermatitis Research Group scoring system as follows:
- NT: Not tested
- –: Negative
- ?+: Doubtful reaction
- +: Weak (nonvesicular) reaction
- ++: Strong (edematous or vesicular) reaction
- +++: Extreme positive reaction
- IR: Irritant reaction of different types

False positive reactions can be seen due to:
- Excessive concentration/amount of allergen
- Impure substance (contaminants)
- Irritant vehicle
- Adhesive tape reactions
- Current dermatitis at the patch-test site or distant site
- "Angry back" reaction
- Artefact

False negative reactions may be because of:
- Insufficient concentration
- Inappropriate vehicle
- Poor adhesion of patches
- Readings taken too early
- Pretreatment of patch test site with topical steroids
- Patient is on immunosuppressants

Angry back reaction: It is also known as the "excited skin syndrome" or "status eczematous". This is a form of hyper-reactivity of the skin of the patch test site because of the presence of any active eczema which renders the whole skin more irritable and thereby causes false positive reactions to allergens and increased reactivity to irritants.

Other types of patch tests:
Open test: In these tests, the liquid test material is applied over skin area of about 1 cm diameter and is allowed to dry. Such reactions may develop sooner and are weaker than a closed patch test reaction. Thus open test is more suitable as a basic screening test for less well-known allergens.

Semi-open test: This kind of test may be used when testing certain emulsifiers, solvents, or other irritant substances.

Photopatch test: It is patch testing followed by irradiation to the test area to cause a photoantigen formation. In one set, the patches are removed after 24 hours and the test site irradiated with 10–15 J/cm^2 of UVA light. The patches are then replaced and the final reading is taken at 48 hours after irradiation. This type of patch test is best suited for patients with history of eczema on the light-exposed site which tend to worsen on exposure of sunlight. Agents causing photocontact dermatitis include fragrances, sunscreens, antibacterial agents, dyes, drugs (sulfonamides, phenothiazines, psoralens, and thiazides) and coal tar derivatives.

Repeat Open Application Test

This test is useful in "doubtful" positive patch test result shown by preparations with low offending allergen concentration. In this test, substances are applied two times a day for 7 days. Upper arm or the flexor surface of the forearm is the most common site of the test.

Thin-layer Rapid Use Epicutaneous Test

It is a prepackaged, ready to use test. It is a convenient, portable method for those who wish to test for a few allergens.

Hematology

Sunita Gupta, Sumit Gupta, Jasleen Kaur, Rohit Batra, Namya Gupta, Meghna Khatri

BLOOD CELLS

Sunita Gupta, Sumit Gupta

INTRODUCTION

Blood accounts for 7% of the body weight, with an average density around 1,060 kg/m^3, which is very close to the density of pure water (1,000 kg/m^3). The average adult has a blood volume of approximately 5 L, which is composed of plasma and several kinds of cells. These blood cells (which are also called corpuscles or "formed elements") consist of erythrocytes [red blood cells (RBCs)], leukocytes [white blood cells (WBCs)] and thrombocytes (platelets). By volume, the RBCs constitute about 45% of whole blood, plasma about 54.3% and white cells about 0.7%.

Blood cells are of three types:
1. Red blood cells
2. *White blood cells*:
   - Granulocytes—neutrophils, eosinophils, and basophils
   - Agranulocytes—lymphocytes and monocytes
3. Platelets

Methods of examination of blood cells:
- Peripheral blood smear—using hematoxylin and eosin (H&E) stain and Romanowsky stain
- Neubauer chamber
- Automated cell counter—four part and six part

RED BLOOD CELLS

- Origin—bone marrow
- Precursor cell—proerythroblast
- Normal count (**Box 1**).

BOX 1	Normal count of blood cells.

- *RBCs*:
  - Males: 4.7–6.1 million cells per microliter
  - Females: 4.2–5.4 million cells per microliter
- *WBCs*: Neutrophils—2,500–8,000 per mm^3 (55–70%):
  - Eosinophils: 50–500 per mm^3 (1–4%)
  - Lymphocytes: 1,000–4,000 per mm^3 (20–40%)
  - Basophils: 25–100 per mm^3 (0.5–1%)
  - Monocytes: 100–700 per mm^3 (2–8%)
- *Platelets*: 150,000–400,000 cells per microliter

(RBC: red blood cell; WBC: white blood cell)

- - Males: 4.7–6.1 million cells per microliter
  - Females: 4.2–5.4 million cells per microliter
- *Red blood cells increased in*: Polycythemia vera, high altitude, after exercise, emotional conditions, smoking and dehydration.
- *Red blood cells decreased in*: Anemia, leukemia, erythropoietin deficiency, hemolytic anemia, chronic renal failure and bone marrow failure.
- *Importance in dermatology*: Sometimes in cases of livedo reticularis, aquagenic pruritus, pyoderma gangrenosum, erythromelalgia and acrocyanosis, RBC count may be increased.

WHITE BLOOD CELLS

Neutrophils

- Origin—bone marrow
- Precursor cell—myeloblast
- Normal count (**Box 1**)—2,500–8,000 per mm^3 (55–70%)
- *Neutrophilia seen in*: Acute infections, metabolic disorders, chronic myeloid leukemia, excessive exercise, high stress levels, poisoning by chemicals and drugs, smoking, chronic inflammation, steroid intake, hyperactive marrow, postsplenectomy and hypoxia
- *Neutropenia seen in*: Autoimmune diseases, tuberculosis (TB), aplastic anemia, sepsis, bone marrow failure, myelodysplastic syndromes, arsenic poisoning, hemodialysis, radiation and chemotherapy
- *Importance in dermatology*: Neutrophils are increased in a variety of skin conditions like Sweet syndrome, pyoderma gangrenosum, Behçet's syndrome, neutrophilic urticarial dermatosis,

dermatitis herpetiformis, psoriasis, hidradenitis suppurativa and subcorneal pustular dermatosis. Neutropenia may be seen in systemic lupus erythematosus (SLE) and poikiloderma.

- They can also rise in cases of prolonged steroid therapy and also in cases of acute skin injuries, drug reactions, erythroderma and Stevens–Johnson syndrome/toxic epidermal necrolysis (SJS/TEN), etc.

Eosinophils

- Origin—bone marrow
- Precursor cell—myeloblast
- Normal count (**Box 1**)—50–500 per mm^3 (1–4%)
- *Eosinophilia seen in*: Parasitic and fungal diseases, allergic reactions such as hay fever and asthma, toxins, autoimmune disorders, endocrine disorders, inflammatory disorders such as coeliac disease and inflammatory bowel disease
- Eosinopenia seen in bacterial infections, stress, prolonged administration of drugs and Cushing syndrome
- *Importance in dermatology*: Eosinophilic dermatoses includes allergic drug eruption, drug-induced erythroderma, urticaria, atopic dermatitis, eczema, allergic contact dermatitis, arthropod bites, and bullous pemphigoid. Eosinophil infiltration is seen in eosinophilic fasciitis, eosinophilic pustular folliculitis and cutaneous eosinophilic vasculitis.

Lymphocytes

- Origin—bone marrow
- Precursor cell—lymphoblast
- Normal count (**Box 1**)—1,000–4,000 per mm^3 (20–40%)
- *Lymphocytosis seen in*: TB, syphilis, malnutrition, acute viral infections such

as chicken pox, herpes, rubella, Epstein–Barr virus (EBV) and cytomegalovirus (CMV) infection, toxoplasmosis, acute lymphocytic leukemia, chronic lymphocytic leukemia, hepatitis A, B, C and hypothyroidism.

- *Lymphocytopenia seen in*: Autoimmune disorders such as rheumatoid arthritis and SLE, radiation and chemotherapy, aplastic anemia, Hodgkin's lymphoma, steroid administration, infections like human immunodeficiency virus (HIV), viral hepatitis, typhoid fever and influenza.
- *Importance in dermatology*: Lymphocytosis is seen in a variety of skin conditions including atopic dermatitis, mycosis fungoides, atopic eczema, psoriasis, subcutaneous panniculitis, Sezary syndrome, pemphigus, alopecia areata, bullous pemphigoid, scleroderma, epidermolysis bullosa acquisita, dermatomyositis, dermatitis herpetiformis and vitiligo. Lymphocytopenia is seen in SLE and leprosy.

Basophils

- Origin—bone marrow
- Precursor cell—myeloblast
- Normal count (**Box 1**)—25-100 per mm^3 (0.5-1%)
- Basophilia seen in infections such as chicken pox, TB, myeloproliferative disorders, chronic hemolytic anemia, allergic reactions, urticaria, food allergy, rheumatoid arthritis and ulcerative colitis
- Basopenia seen in stress, exposure to chemotherapy or radiation therapy and hypersensitivity reactions.
- *Importance in dermatology*: Basopenia is seen in chronic urticaria. Basophils are seen in prurigo, insect bite reaction, drug eruptions, Henoch–Schönlein purpura, scabies and bullous pemphigoid.

Monocytes

- Origin—bone marrow
- Precursor cell—monoblast
- Normal count (**Box 1**)—100-700 per mm^3 (2-8%)
- Monocytosis seen in infections such as TB, malaria, kala-azar, myeloproliferative disorders, obesity, malignancies like Hodgkin's lymphoma, rheumatoid arthritis and monocytic or myelomonocytic leukemia
- Monocytopenia seen in prolonged use of glucocorticoids, acute infections, aplastic anemia, acute myeloid leukemia, bone marrow failure and hairy cell leukemia
- *Importance in dermatology*: Monocytes are seen in a variety of skin conditions such as psoriasis, atopic dermatitis, SLE, Sezary syndrome, herpes zoster and leprosy

Platelets

- Origin—bone marrow
- Precursor cell—megakaryoblast
- *Normal count (**Box 1**)*: 1,50,000-4,00,000 cells per microliter
- Thrombocytosis is seen in high altitude, allergic conditions, splenectomy, trauma, chronic inflammation, iron deficiency, acute blood loss, essential thrombocytosis, inflammatory bowel disease, rheumatoid arthritis, nephrotic syndrome, bacterial diseases including sepsis, pneumonia, meningitis and urinary tract infections.
- Thrombocytopenia is seen in splenomegaly, chicken pox, aplastic and pernicious anemia, acute leukemia, TB, radiotherapy and chemotherapy, HELLP syndrome (hemolysis, elevated liver enzymes and low platelet), hemolytic uremic syndrome, familial thrombocytopenia, immune and thrombotic thrombocytopenic purpura, cirrhosis,

heparin-induced thrombocytopenia, dengue and babesiosis.

- *Importance in dermatology*: Role and importance of platelets has been described in skin lesions of hemangioma, vasculitis, eczema, SLE, dengue fever, postviral exanthem, Wiskott–Aldrich syndrome, atopic dermatitis, contact dermatitis, urticaria, psoriasis, idiopathic thrombocytopenic purpura (ITP) and preparation of platelet rich plasma.

RED CELL INDICES

Sumit Gupta, Jasleen Kaur

INTRODUCTION

These are different blood tests which provide indirect information about the hemoglobin (Hb) level and RBC size. Abnormal values of red cell indices may indicate the presence and type of anemia.

Types

Different red cell indices are:

- Mean corpuscular hemoglobin (MCH)
- Mean corpuscular volume (MCV)
- Mean corpuscular hemoglobin concentration (MCHC)
- Red cell distribution width

Mean corpuscular volume: MCV is a measure of the average volume of a RBC.

Mean corpuscular volume is calculated by: MCV = PCV/RBC count × 100

MCV normal value is 80–100 fl (femtoliter) of normocytic RBC's

So, if value is <80 fl = Microcytic RBC's

>100 = Macrocytic RBC's (**Table 1**)

Mean corpuscular hemoglobin: MCH is average mass of Hb per RBC in a sample of blood.

MCH = Hb/RBC × 10

Normal value is = 27–32 pg (picogram)

If MCH value is <27 pg = RBC's hypochromic

>27 pg = RBC's hyperchromic (**Table 2**)

Mean corpuscular hemoglobin concentration: MCHC is measure of the concentration of Hb in a given volume of packed RBC (**Table 3**).

MCHC is calculated by: Hb/PCV × 10

where, Hb is hemoglobin; PCV is packed cell volume

MCHC normal value is 32–36 g/dL

TABLE 1: Causes of alteration in MCV levels.		
MCV increased (macrocytic RBCs)	**MCV decreased (microcytic RBCs)**	**MCV normal (normocytic RBCs)**
Pernicious anemia	Iron deficiency anemia (IDA)	Early IDA
Vitamin B12 or folic acid deficiency	Beta-thalassemia	Hemorrhage
Chronic lymphocytic leukemia	Anemia of chronic disease	Renal failure
Hypothyroidism	Lead poisoning	Primary marrow disorders
Myelodysplastic syndrome		Aplastic anemia
Bone marrow failure (aplastic anemia)		

(MCV: mean corpuscular volume; RBCs: red blood cells)

TABLE 2: Causes of alteration in MCH level.	
MCH increased	**MCH decreased**
Polycythemia	Iron deficiency anemia
Liver disease	Celiac disease causing nutritional deficiencies
Estrogen intake	
Chronic alcoholic	

(MCH: mean corpuscular hemoglobin)

TABLE 3: Causes of alteration in MCHC levels.	
MCHC increased	**MCHC decreased**
Hereditary spherocytosis	Microcytic—iron deficiency
Sickle cell anemia	
Autoimmune hemolytic anemia	
Macrocytic anemia	
Severe burns	
Spherocytosis due to any cause	

(MCHC: mean corpuscular hemoglobin concentration)

Red cell distribution width: RBC distribution width (RDW or RDW-CV or RCDW and RDW-SD) is a measure of the range of variation of volume of RBC. Usually RBCs have a standard size of about 6–8 µm in diameter. Certain disorders can cause a significant variation in cell size. Higher RDW values indicate greater variation in size. RDW test results are often used together with MCV results in cases of anemia to determine the possible cause. It is mainly used to differentiate an anemia of mixed causes from an anemia of a single cause.

The RDW is calculated with the following formula:
- RDW–CV = (Standard deviation of MCV ÷ MCV) × 100

Normal reference range of RDW in human RBCs is 11.5–15.4%.

Normal RDW: Anemia in the presence of a normal RDW may suggest thalassemia or anemia of chronic diseases.

High RDW: High RDW may be a result of the presence of fragments, groups of agglutination, and/or abnormal shape of RBCs:
- Iron-deficiency anemia usually presents with high RDW and low MCV.
- Folate and vitamin B-12 deficiency anemia usually present with high RDW and high MCV.
- Mixed-deficiency (iron + B12 or folate) anemia usually presents with high RDW and variable MCV.
- Recent hemorrhages typically present with high RDW and normal MCV.
- A false high RDW reading can occur, if ethylene diamine tetra acetic acid (EDTA)-anticoagulated blood is used instead of citrated blood.

HEMOGLOBIN

Rohit Batra, Namya Gupta

INTRODUCTION

Hemoglobin is an oxygen-binding protein found in RBCs which transports oxygen from the lungs to tissues.

Each Hb molecule is a tetramer made of four polypeptide globin chains. Each globin subunit contains a heme moiety formed of an organic protoporphyrin ring and a central iron ion in the ferrous state (Fe^{2+}).

The iron molecule in each heme moiety can bind and unbind oxygen, allowing for oxygen transport in the body. The most common type of Hb in the adult is HbA, which comprises two alpha-globin and two beta-globin subunits. The fetal and infantile Hb is composed of two alpha and gamma chains each. There is no beta chain at this age. As the child grows the gamma chains are replaced by beta chains forming adult Hb.

The iron content in Hb gives red color to RBCs. It also helps in maintenance of shape of RBCs. So the abnormal Hb causes disruption of shape of RBCs which leads to dysfunction and hemolysis.

Measurement of hemoglobin: There are several methods of measurement of Hb but due to technological advancement, nowadays it is done in automated machines.

In the machine, RBCs are broken down which releases Hb and this free Hb is exposed to some chemicals containing cyanide and make cyanomethemoglobin. Then a special light is passed through the solution and the amount of light absorbed and reflected at a particular wavelength of 540 nm indicates the Hb amount.

SAHLI'S METHOD

Sahli's hemoglobinometer is a manual device that contains a Hb tube, pipette and stirrer, as well as a comparator. Hydrochloric acid converts Hb to acid hematin, which is then diluted until the color of the solution matches that of the comparator block.

The technician can then ascertain the Hb concentration by reading from the calibration tube. This is one of the most common methods for estimating Hb in developing countries. It is relatively simple and inexpensive but the results are not always precise, as there is often inter-observer variability and it is highly prone to errors due to manual pipetting.

Normal levels:
- *Newborns*: 17–22 g/dL
- *1 week of age*: 15–20 g/dL
- *1 month of age*: 11–15 g/dL
- *Children*: 11–13 g/dL
- *Adult males*: 14–18 g/dL
- *Adult women*: 12–16 g/dL
- *Men after middle age*: 12.4–14.9 g/dL
- *Women after middle age*: 11.7–13.8 g/dL

Anemia

Anemia is a medical condition in which the RBC count or Hb is less than normal. Symptoms of anemia include:
- Fatigue
- Feeling of unwellness
- Heart palpitations
- Shortness of breath

Some of the more common causes of anemia are:
- Loss of blood (traumatic injury, surgery, bleeding, colon cancer, or stomach ulcer)
- Nutritional deficiency (iron, vitamin B12, and folate)
- Bone marrow dysfunction due to drugs, leukemia, viral infections, etc.
- Suppression by RBC synthesis by chemotherapy drugs, Kidney failure, etc.
- Abnormal Hb structure like in thalassemia or sickle cell anemia.

How to increase Hb?
- Red blood cell transfusion and injection erythropoietin (commonly used in cases of chronic renal failure)
- Taking iron supplements
- Intake of iron-rich foods, e.g., green leafy vegetables, seafood, eggs, beans, etc.
- Intake of foods rich in cofactors such as vitamin B6, B12, C and folic acid, e.g., seafood, green leafy vegetables, cereals, nuts, and citrus fruits, etc.

Abnormally high levels of Hb are seen in smokers and people living at high altitudes. In intensive care unit (ICU), trauma patients can also show high Hb because of hemoconcentration, if proper hydration is not maintained.

Some other infrequent causes of high Hb levels are:
- Advanced lung disease (e.g., emphysema);
- Certain tumors.
- A disorder of the bone marrow known as polycythemia rubra vera.
- Abuse of the drug erythropoietin (Epogen) by athletes for blood doping purposes (increases the amount of oxygen available to the body by chemically raising the production of RBCs).

Importance in dermatology: Skin is an accessory organ having the largest surface area. In case of any type of anemia, skin is the first organ to be deprived of proper nutrition and waste disposal. So, first signs of any kind of deficiency or anemia appears in the skin.

Nutritional Anemia

Anemia can be the result of nutrient deficiencies, e.g., iron, B12 or folate.

Skin manifestations are:
- Pallor of the conjunctiva (eyes) and palmar creases
- Glossitis (smooth red tongue)
- Poikilodermatous hypopigmentation
- Hyperpigmentation may be a sign of B12 and folate deficiencies
- Brittle nails (koilonychia)

Hemolytic anemia leads to additional symptoms such as:
- Pruritus
- Jaundice
- Petechiae and hemosiderosis (small brown macules)

Polycythemia vera is an example of a chronic myeloproliferative disorder of myeloid cells that results in an increased red cell mass.

Skin manifestations of Polycythemia vera are:
- Plethora/ruddy cyanosis (florid complexion)
- Aquagenic pruritus (itching of skin triggered by contact with water)
- Erythromelalgia (redness and burning pain of hands/feet)
- Livedo reticularis (purplish lace-like discoloration)
- Acrocyanosis (bluish-purplish discoloration of hands/feet)
- Pyoderma gangrenosum (ulcers)

Various other disorders like lymphoproliferative disorders, coagulation disorders can present with specific skin lesions along with abnormality in cell counts and morphology.

ERYTHROCYTE SEDIMENTATION RATE

Sumit Gupta, Meghna Khatri

INTRODUCTION

An erythrocyte sedimentation rate (ESR) is a blood test that measures how quickly erythrocytes (RBCs) settle at the bottom of a test tube. Normally, erythrocytes settle relatively slowly. A faster rate may indicate presence of inflammatory process in the body. It can be a reaction to an infection or injury. Inflammation may also be a sign of a chronic disease, an immune disorder or other medical condition.

Erythrocyte sedimentation rate is a nonspecific measure of inflammation. The ESR is governed by the balance between pro sedimentation factors, mainly fibrinogen and those factors resisting sedimentation, namely the negative charge of the erythrocytes (zeta potential). When an inflammatory process is present, the high proportion of fibrinogen in the blood causes RBCs to stick to each other. The red cells form stacks called rouleaux which settle faster due to their increased density.

Erythrocyte sedimentation rate is the measure of ability of erythrocytes to fall through the blood plasma and accumulate together at the base of container at the end of 1 hour.

There are three stages in erythrocyte sedimentation:
1. Rouleaux formation
2. Sedimentation or settling stage
3. Packing stage—10 minutes (sedimentation slows and cells start to pack at the bottom of the tube)

Measurement of ESR: ESR can be measured by a variety of methods, including the

Westergren, Wintrobe and micro-ESR, along with the use of automated machines.

Westergren Method

The Westergren method has classically been used to measure the ESR. It is based on the distance that RBCs settle to the bottom of an elongated tube with a 2.5 cm internal bore. It is graduated downward in millimeters (0–200 mm), it allows the clear plasma to remain at the top of the tube, after the sedimentation of RBCs at the bottom due to gravitational force after 1 hour of observation.

Normal values for the ESR, as obtained using the Westergren method, are as follows:
- Male < 50 years ≤ 15 mm/h
- Female < 50 years ≤ 20 mm/h
- Male > 50 years ≤ 20 mm/h
- Female > 50 years ≤ 30 mm/h
- Child ≤ 10 mm/h

The ESR is typically higher in females than in males and increases gradually with age.

The method is time consuming and there is also chances of manual error, so newer methods of measuring ESR have evolved.

Micro Erythrocyte Sedimentation Rate

The micro ESR is a method of obtaining the ESR using capillary tubes and is relatively quicker method. This method uses four drops of capillary blood drawn from a finger prick which is then mixed with a 3.8% sodium citrate solution in a ratio of 4:1 on a slide. The sample is then drawn into a 7.5-cm heparin-free microhematocrit capillary tube. The results are measured after just 20 minutes and then adjusted to predict conventional ESR values from the micro ESR value.

Several new automated and semiautomated techniques have become available for determining the ESR that are safer and faster with a higher level of accuracy.

Clinical Importance

Several factors may influence the ESR:
- Females tend to have slightly increased ESRs compared to males.
- Pregnancy and aging may also increase the ESR.
- Anemia, RBC abnormalities, technical factors such as tilted ESR tubes, increased temperature of the specimen, and dilution errors may increase the ESR.

Erythrocyte sedimentation rate is a very misleading/inconclusive test which is neither specific nor sensitive though it is done routinely as a screening test. The high ESR gives a suspicion of some underlying pathology. The different causes of high ESR are as below:
- Anemia
- Arteritis
- Infections (including bone and joint)
- Kidney disease
- Low serum albumin
- Lupus
- Lymphoma
- Multiple myeloma
- Polymyalgia rheumatica
- Red blood cell abnormalities
- Rheumatoid arthritis
- Systemic vasculitis
- Thyroid disease
- Waldenstrom macroglobulinemia

The ESR is decreased in:
- Polycythemia, hyper viscosity, sickle cell anemia, leukemia, chronic fatigue syndrome, low plasma protein (due to liver or kidney disease) and congestive heart failure.
- Although raised levels of immunoglobulins usually increase the ESR, very high levels of the same can reduce the ESR due to hyper viscosity of the plasma.

- Regular intake of alcohol may lead to lowering of ESR.
- Regular heavy and moderate physical exercise can lead to low ESR.

RETICULOCYTE COUNT

Sumit Gupta, Rohit Batra

INTRODUCTION

Reticulocytes are immature RBCs produced in the bone marrow and released into the peripheral blood where they mature into RBCs within 1–2 days.

An increase or decrease in reticulocyte count can be an indicator of erythropoiesis activity or failure, especially relative to anemias and bone marrow dysfunction.

A normal reticulocyte count for healthy adults who are not anemic is around 0.5–2.5%.

A high reticulocyte count may indicate:
- Anemia due to RBCs being destroyed earlier than normal (hemolytic anemia)
- Bleeding
- Blood disorder in a fetus or newborn (erythroblastosis fetalis)
- Kidney disease with increased production of a hormone called erythropoietin
- Reticulocyte count may be higher during pregnancy

A low reticulocyte count may indicate:
- Hypochromic anemias-because of the decreased Hb synthesis in these type of anemias. For example thalassemia, iron deficiency anemia, anemia of chronic disease, sideroblastic anemia, etc.
- Nutritional deficiency anemias such as megaloblastic anemia which occur due to the deficiency of vitamin B12 and folic acid. There is a decreased synthesis of DNA in bone marrow which in turn leads to decreased production of reticulocytes.
- Hemolytic anemia with aplastic crisis—Usually patients with hemolytic anemias present with increased retic count but in some cases they can have decreased retic count which can be due to aplastic crisis. It represents a temporary decrease in the process of erythropoiesis due to unavailability or insufficient amounts of cellular precursors in bone marrow. Probable cause is mostly an infection due to organisms like salmonella, parvovirus B19 and *Streptococcus pneumoniae*.
- *Myelodysplastic syndromes*: These syndromes can present with damage to the bone marrow due to multiple causes which can affect the erythropoietic cell line leading to decreased reticulocyte count.
- Failure of bone marrow due to various causes such as drugs, radiation therapy, infection or malignancy.
- Cirrhosis of the liver
- Chronic kidney disease

Importance in Dermatology

Routinely advised in patients on dapsone therapy for estimation of extent of hemolysis.

Blood Glucose

Sunita Gupta, Sanjeev Gupta

INTRODUCTION

The blood sugar or blood glucose level is the concentration of glucose present in the blood. Glucose is a simple sugar and approximately 4–5 g of glucose is present in the blood of a 70-kg adult at all times. If we take the blood volume of 5 L, a blood glucose level of 5.5 mmol/L (100 mg/dL) amounts to 5 g, equivalent to about a teaspoonful of sugar.

According to American Diabetes Association (ADA) guidelines:
- Fasting plasma glucose level—100–125 mg/dL-impaired, 126 mg or more falls into the diabetic range.
- Postprandial level—140–199 mg/dL-impaired, 200 mg or more falls into the diabetic range.

BLOOD GLUCOSE

- The target level of normal blood glucose level (tested while fasting):
  - For nondiabetics 70–100 mg/dL
  - For diabetics 80–130 mg/dL
- Despite widely variable intervals between meals, human blood glucose levels tend to remain within the normal range. However, immediately after food intake, the blood glucose level may rise in non-diabetics temporarily up to 140 mg/dL or slightly more.
- In patients with diabetes, for maintaining "tight diabetes control", the ADA recommends a peak postprandial glucose level of <10 mmol/L (180 mg/dL)

Note:
- Sample collection is a very important step in case of indoor patients, especially when patient is on IV fluids/glucose. If sample is collected from same limb, while infusion is on, it will alter glucose level. So to prevent it, sample to be taken from other limb or 5–10 minutes after the infusion has been stopped. Suppose patient is on 5% dextrose, even the 10% contamination of sample can lead to rise in blood glucose as high as 500 mg/dL.
- There is slight variation in arterial/venous and capillary blood glucose in random state. But postmeal glucose level is higher in arterial and capillary than venous sample.
- The mean capillary glucose is usually higher than the mean venous blood concentration, difference may be as high as 35%.

- The mean glucose level varies in whole blood, plasma and serum.
- Earlier, blood glucose level was measured in whole blood, but now a days, most of the laboratories estimate glucose in plasma or serum. Serum and plasma have higher glucose level than whole blood because of more water content. A multiplication factor of 1.14 is used to convert whole blood sample reading to serum level.

Causes of abnormal blood glucose:
- *Reference range. Fasting blood glucose (FBG)*: 70–100 mg/dL as per ADA guidelines
- *Persistent hyperglycemia*: Diabetes mellitus, adrenal cortical hyperactivity Cushing's syndrome, hyperthyroidism, acromegaly and obesity
- *Transient hyperglycemia*: Pheochromocytoma, severe liver disease, acute stress reaction, shock and convulsions
- *Persistent hypoglycemia*: Insulinoma, adrenal cortical inefficiency, Addison's disease, hypopituitarism, galactosemia and ectopic insulin production from tumors.
- *Transient hypoglycemia*: Acute alcohol ingestion, drugs like salicylates, antitubercular drugs, severe liver disease, several glycogen storage diseases and hereditary fructose intolerance.

DRUGS CAUSING HYPERGLYCEMIA

- Corticosteroids
- Octreotide
- Beta blocker
- Statins
- Thiazides
- Niacin
- Diuretics
- Antipsychotics
- Cyclosporine

ORAL GLUCOSE TOLERANCE TEST

During a glucose tolerance test (GTT), which may be used to diagnose diabetes mellitus, a fasting patient takes a 75 g oral glucose. Then blood glucose levels are measured after 2 hours.

Interpretation is based on WHO guidelines:
- After 2 hours, a glycemia < 7.8 mmol/L (140 mg/dL) is considered normal.
- A glycemia of between 7.8 and 11.0 mmol/L (140–197 mg/dL) is considered as impaired glucose tolerance (IGT) and
- A glycemia of ≥11.1 mmol/L (200 mg/dL) is considered diabetes mellitus.
  An oral glucose tolerance test (OGTT) may be normal or mildly abnormal in simple insulin resistance.

Importance in Dermatology
- Most of our patients receive systemic steroids which causes hyperglycemia, so monitoring is very important.
- Many patients receive immunosuppressants and immunomodulators (Cyclosporine), so baseline blood sugar is important in such cases, as underlying impaired glucose level may increase the risk of infections.
- Blood glucose may transiently rise in cases of stress, especially in cases of skin injury, inflammatory conditions like Stevens–Johnson syndrome (SJS), toxic epidermal necrolysis (TEN), erythroderma, etc.

Glycosylated Hemoglobin

Sunita Gupta, Sanjeev Gupta

INTRODUCTION

Glycosylated hemoglobin or glyco hemoglobin (HbA1c, hemoglobin A1c, A1c or less commonly HbA1c, HgbA1c, Hb1c, etc.) is a form of hemoglobin that is chemically linked to a sugar. Red blood cells live for 3 months, so this test shows the average level of glucose in your blood for the past 3 months.

Adult hemoglobin is made up of three different forms of Hb namely: HbA1, HbA2, HbF. Out of these HbA1 predominates and consists of three subforms namely: HbA1a, HbA1b and HbA1c, out of these HbA1c predominates.

The term glycation or glycosylation means attachment of sugar molecules with Hb, which is an irreversible process. Once the sugar molecules enter RBC and attach with Hb molecule, it cannot be detached until RBC is hemolysed.

The high levels of HbA1c diffuses through vessel wall and binds with nitric oxide which is otherwise needed for acetylcholine—induced endothelium-dependent relaxation and so, causing prevention of its normal function. This in turn may lead to vessel damage, narrowing and atherogenic plaque formation.

The 2010 American Diabetes Association Standards of Medical Care in Diabetes added the HbA1c $\geq$ 48 mmol/mol ($\geq$6.5%) as another criterion for the diagnosis of diabetes.

Normal ranges for HbA1c:
- <5.7 = Normal
- 5.7–6.4 = Prediabetic
- >6.5 = Diabetic
- HbA1c values can help in determining the mean plasma glucose levels of the patient (**Table 1**).

Important notes:
- *Hemolytic anemia* decreases HbA1c levels because of increased production of

TABLE 1: HbA1c and corresponding mean plasma glucose levels.	
HbA1c (%)	**Mean plasma glucose (mg/dL)**
6	126
7	154
8	183
9	212
10	240
11	269
12	298

(HbA1c: glycosylated hemoglobin)

younger red blood cells, which contains hemoglobin with less exposure to ambient glycemia.

- Aplastic and/or iron deficiency anemia increases the average age of circulating erythrocytes, leading to increased concentration of HbA1c independent of glycemia.
- The HbA1c level is increased by approximately 0.1% with a decrease of 2 g/dL in the hemoglobin level at the same fasting glucose level in people without anemia. Therefore, for HbA1c to be reliable, the patient should not be anemic.

CONDITIONS CAUSING FALSE HIGH/LOW HbA1c LEVELS

- Conditions causing inappropriately low HbA1c are hemoglobinopathies and hemolytic disease, pregnancy, blood transfusion, hypertriglyceridemia, acute blood loss, drugs and chronic liver disease
- Conditions causing inappropriately high HbA1c—iron deficiency, vitamin B12 deficiency, uremia, alcoholism and hyperbilirubinemia
- Variable effect on HbA1c—fetal hemoglobin and methemoglobin

DRUGS CAUSING INAPPROPRIATELY LOW OR HIGH HbA1c

Falsely low levels of HbA1c:
- Due to increased erythrocyte destruction—dapsone, ribavirin and trimethoprim-sulfamethoxazole, etc.

- Due to altered hemoglobin—hydroxyurea
- Due to altered glycation—vitamin A, vitamin C and aspirin in low doses

Falsely high levels of HbA1c: Caused due to interference with assays opiates, aspirin in high doses.

Methods of measuring HbA1c:
- Iron exchange chromatography: High-performance liquid chromatography (HPLC)
- Electrophoretic methods
- Immunoturbidimetric methods
- Chemical methods
- Mass spectroscopy

The mean plasma glucose (MPG) can be calculated by HbA1c by following formula:

$$MPG = (33.3 \times HbA1c\%) - 86$$

Current uses of HbA1c:
- Diagnosis of diabetes
- Monitor long-term glycemic control
- Adjustment or titration of dosage for better control of blood glucose
- Predict the risk of development of complications

Glycosylated hemoglobin correlates directly with retinopathy. The glycemic levels at which prevalence of retinopathy begins to rise above the rest of the population is around 6.5%.

Importance in Dermatology

- Multiple studies have shown a linear relationship between HbA1c and dyslipidemia.
- HbA1c values can be of diagnostic and prognostic significance in patients with dyslipidemic and diabetic skin complications.

Urine Examination

Aneet Mahendra, Sanjeev Gupta

INTRODUCTION

Urine examination is a very simple, economical and easily available basic investigation which may be very useful for the detection and management of wide range of disorders especially renal diseases, urinary tract infection, diabetes, etc., though it can also be inconclusive many a times.

- There are three basic components to urinalysis which include gross examination, chemical and microscopic examination.
- The container for urine collection should be clean, wide open mouth, dry and the sample should be analyzed within 1–2 hours or should be refrigerated.

Gross examination: Volume, color, transparency, odor, specific gravity and pH.

Most of components in urinalysis can be estimated by urine test strips (in dipstick method, the color should be matched as per the prescribed time strictly, otherwise the color will derange and will give false reading), light microscopic examination is done after centrifugation of sample to see RBC, WBC, epithelial cells, casts, mucus, pus cells, bacteria, fungus, calcium oxalate crystals, etc.

pH: pH of urine may vary from 4.5 to 8, usually it is acidic in range of 6–6.5.

- High acidic pH may be because of ketosis, fever, starvation and *Escherichia coli* infection.
- Increase in alkalinity of urine can be due to:
  - Urinary tract infection (*Proteus* and others);
  - Metabolic alkalosis (pyloric stenosis and others);
  - Failure of acidification (renal tubular acidosis, chronic renal failure or aldosterone abnormalities);
  - Ingestion (salicylate, sodium bicarbonate, acetazolamide, etc.); and
  - Respiratory alkalosis (hyperventilation)

Color: Normal urine color may vary as per hydration status of patient and may vary as per diet and drug intake.

- *Nearly colorless*: Excessive fluid intake for conditions; untreated diabetes mellitus, diabetes insipidus and certain types of nephritis.
- *Yellow*: Distinctly yellow urine may indicate excessive riboflavin (vitamin B2) intake.
- *Yellow-amber*: Normal
- *Yellow-cloudy*: Excessive crystals (crystalluria) and/or excessive pus (pyuria).

- *Orange*: Insufficient fluid intake for conditions; intake of orange substances; intake of phenazopyridine for urinary symptoms.
- *Red*: Leakage of red blood cells and intake of red substances.
- *Dark*:
  - Reddish-orange: Intake of certain medications or other substances.
  - Rusty-yellow to reddish-brown: Intake of certain medications or other substances.
  - Dark brown: Intake of certain medications or other substances; damaged muscle (myoglobinuria due to rhabdomyolysis) from extreme exercise or other widespread damage, possibly medication related; altered blood; bilirubinuria; intake of phenolic substances; inadequate porphyrin metabolism; melanin from melanocytic tumors; presence of an abnormal form of hemoglobin and methemoglobin.
  - Brownish-black to black: Intake of substances or medications; altered blood; a problem with homogentisic acid metabolism (alkaptonuria), which can also cause darkening of the sclera and dark-colored internal structures (ochronosis); lysol (a product that contains phenols) poisoning; melanin (from melanocytic tumors). Paraphenylenediamine is a highly toxic ingredient of hair dye formulations that can cause acute kidney injury and result in black urine.
  - Purple due to purple urine bag syndrome.
- *Magenta to purple-red*: Presence of phenolphthalein
- *Green or dark with a greenish hue*: Jaundice (bilirubinuria); problem with bile metabolism, high doses of propofol infusion.
- *Milky white*: Presence of fat globules (chyluria) due to filariasis.
- *Other colors*: Various substances ingested in food or drink, particularly up to 48 hours prior to the presence of colored urine.

AMOUNT

Causes of excess urine volume include:
- Bladder infection (common in children and women)
- Type 1 and type 2 diabetes mellitus
- Pregnancy
- *Kidney disease or failure*: Damaged kidneys cannot concentrate or process urine. Polyuria can often be an early sign of kidney trouble.
- *Cushing's syndrome*: High cortisol in your body. The extra cortisol affects ADH (antidiuretic hormone), a hormone involved in urine production.
- *Hypercalcemia*: High calcium in blood can affect ADH levels or your kidneys' response to it. It can also affect the way your kidneys process urine.
- *Anxiety*: There's a link between anxiety and vasopressin (this helps kidneys hold onto water).
- *Medications like*:
  - Calcium channel blockers: Vasodilatation caused by these drugs can lead to increased urine output.
  - Diuretics
  - Lithium: Causes damage to kidneys.
  - SSRIs: Used to treat depression but can prevent from making ADH.
  - Tetracycline: Demeclocycline, a form of this antibiotic, can affect ADH production.

- Psychogenic polydipsia, a mental disorder causing excessive thirst.
- Consumption of alcohol or caffeine.

Causes of decreased urine output:
- Dehydration—most common cause of decreased urine output. It can be due to excess diarrhea, vomiting or any other cause of acute fluid loss.
- Infection or trauma—these are less typical causes of oliguria.
- Urinary tract obstruction or blockage—usually results in a decreased urine output because of kidney damage.
- Medications—medicines that are known to possibly cause, this includes:
  - Nonsteroidal anti-inflammatory drugs (NSAIDs)
  - High blood pressure medications such as angiotensin-converting enzyme (ACE) inhibitors
  - Gentamicin

Specific gravity of urine:
- Adults generally have a specific gravity in the range of 1.010–1.030.
- Increase in specific gravity (hypersthenuria, i.e., increased concentration of solutes in the urine) may be associated with dehydration, diarrhea, emesis, excessive sweating, urinary tract/bladder infection, glucosuria, renal artery stenosis, hepatorenal syndrome, decreased blood flow to the kidney (heart failure) and an excess of ADH caused by the syndrome of inappropriate ADH secretion.
- A specific gravity ≥ 1.035 is consistent with frank dehydration.
- In neonates, normal urine specific gravity is 1.003. Hypovolemic patients usually have a specific gravity >1.015.
- Decreased specific gravity (hyposthenuria, i.e., decreased concentration of solutes in urine) may be associated with renal failure, pyelonephritis, diabetes insipidus, acute tubular necrosis, interstitial nephritis and excessive fluid intake (e.g., psychogenic polydipsia).

Odor: It may vary as per hydration status, diet. ketoacidosis in diabetics may have fruity or sweet odor. Foul offensive odor may indicate infection.

Urinary electrolytes:
- *Sodium (Na$^+$)*: Needed for workup of acute renal injury.
- *Potassium (K$^+$)*: It is needed for workup of hypokalemia. If K$^+$ is lost through GIT, the urine K$^+$ will be low, if it is lost through kidney, K$^+$ in urine may be high. Decreased levels of urine K$^+$ are also seen in hypoaldosteronism and adrenal insufficiency.
- *Calcium*: High calcium in urine is called hypercalciuria which may be due to hypercalcemia (hyperparathyroidism, sarcoidosis, other granulomatous diseases, vitamin D intoxication and paraneoplastic syndromes) or even may be with normal serum calcium (renal tubular acidosis, glucocorticoid excess, diuretics and idiopathic).
- *Nitrites*: The presence of nitrites in urine, termed nitrituria may indicate the presence of coliform bacteria.
- *Phosphates*: High phosphate in the urine phosphaturia.
- Primary hyperphosphaturia is because of disorder in kidney, while secondary causes include both types of hyperparathyroidism.

Urine Microscopy

Microscopic examination:
- *Red blood cells*: 0–3/HPF normal.
  - On gross examination urine may be cloudy, red in color.

- It may be due to early glomerular disease, trauma, acute infection, coagulation disorders, malignancy, calculi, strenuous exercise.
  - Hematuria + pyuria/bacteuria = urinary tract infection.
  - Hematuria + RBC casts/dysmorphic RBC + proteinuria = glomerulonephrits
- *White blood cells*: Normal ≤5/hpf, more in females
  - May enter through glomerulus or trauma but also by amoeboid migration
  - Increased WBCs in urine is known as pyuria, it can be due to infectious or sterile cause.
  - Infections: Cystitis, pyelonephritis, prostatitis, urethritis, glomerulonephritis (lupus erythematosus, interstitial nephritis), tumors
  - Sterile pyuria: WBCs in urine but culture is sterile
  - Reports presence or absence of bacteria.
- *Casts*: There are many types of casts, e.g., WBC casts, RBC casts, epithelial casts, bacterial casts and fatty casts.
  - It may be because of nonpathological and pathological causes.
  - Nonpathological causes: stress, heavy exercise, heat exposure, dehydration, fever.
  - Pathological causes: Chronic renal disease, glomerulonephritis, pyelonephritis, congestive heart failure.
- *Epithelial cells are of three types*:
  - i. Squamous: Vagina, male and female urethra
  - ii. Transitional: Bladder, renal pelvis, calyces, ureters, upper male urethra
  - iii. Renal tubular epithelial (RTE) cells: Renal tubules

- *Bacteria*: WBCs can accompany bacteria in UTI
- *Parasites*: Schistosomiasis, enterobius vermicularis
- *Yeast*: Seen in Diabetic urine, as increase in blood glucose leads to increased yeast growth. Also present in patients with immunocompromised status, vaginal candidiasis.
- *Spermatozoa*: It has lack of clinical significance, present in cases with retrograde ejaculation.
- *Crystals*: Uric acid crystals, calcium oxalate crystals, cholesterol crystals, etc.
- *Artifacts*: Material fibers, hair, diaper fibers

Glucose: Refer **Table 1**

TABLE 1: Interpretation of dipstick test for glucosuria.

Urine dipstick designation	Approximate plasma concentration
Trace	100 mg/dL
1+	250 mg/dL
2+	500 mg/dL
3+	1,000 mg/dL
4+	2,000 mg/dL

Proteins: Normally a very minimal amount of protein is lost in urine, which may remain undetected by dipstick method (**Table 2**).

TABLE 2: Interpretation of dipstick test for proteinuria.

Dipstick reading	Protein excretion in mg/dL	Protein excretion in g/24 h
Trace	5–20 mg/dL	0.1–0.2 g/day
1+	30–100 mg/dL	0.2–0.5 g/day
2+	100–300 mg/dL	0.5–1 g/day
3+	300–1,000 mg/dL	1–2 g/day
4+	>1,000 mg/dL	>2 g/day

URINE EXAMINATION AND DERMATOLOGY

- *Urine pregnancy test*: For starting any immunosuppressive treatment or retinoids
- In workup of connective tissue disorders
- In case of diabetic patients
- *Proteinuria* can be a side effect of cyclosporine
- *Microscopic hematuria* in patients taking cyclophosphamide

- Evaluation in cases of urethral discharge [sexually transmitted disease (STD)]
- In cases of skin failure [pemphigus, erythroderma and toxic epidermal necrolysis (TEN)]:
  - In cases of porphyria
  - Workup of a case of retrograde ejaculation
  - Compliance marker of rifampicin (orange colored urine)

Urinary Protein

Sanjeev Gupta, Aneet Mahendra

INTRODUCTION

- Presence of protein in urine is called proteinuria.
- Urine protein (UP) testing is routinely done in routine urine examination by dipstick method.
- It is an important marker of renal disease and used for monitoring, screening, and evaluation of renal disease.
- Presence of significant amount of protein by dipstick methods warns to go for quantitative estimation of UP in 24 hours urine sample.
- Sometimes urinary protein to creatinine ratio (UP/C ratio) is needed in case of massive proteinuria.
- There are some diurnal variations in amount of protein excreted and that too keep changing with age. But that amount is transient and not high.
- Either a 24-hour UP or a random protein to creatinine ratio may be used to monitor a person with known kidney disease or damage. A dipstick UP and/or a protein to creatinine ratio may be used to screen people on a regular basis when they are taking a medication that may affect their kidney function.

SAMPLE COLLECTION

- A single urine sample is collected in a clean container at any time (random/ spot).
- 24-hour urine should be collected by instructing the patient to discard first morning void; specimen of all subsequent voiding should be collected including the first morning sample on second day.
- The sample must be refrigerated preferably during this period or kept in cool and dark place.

Testing Methods

- Heat coagulation test
- Hellers nitric test
- Sulfosalicylic acid test

Interpretation of tests:

- Normal proteinuria is <150 mg/day and <30 mg of albumin/day.

    Sometimes, proteinuria may be temporary because of an infection, medication, heavy exercise, high protein diet, severe stress, pregnancy, and cold exposure.
- Diabetes and hypertension are two main causes of persistent proteinuria in clinical practice.

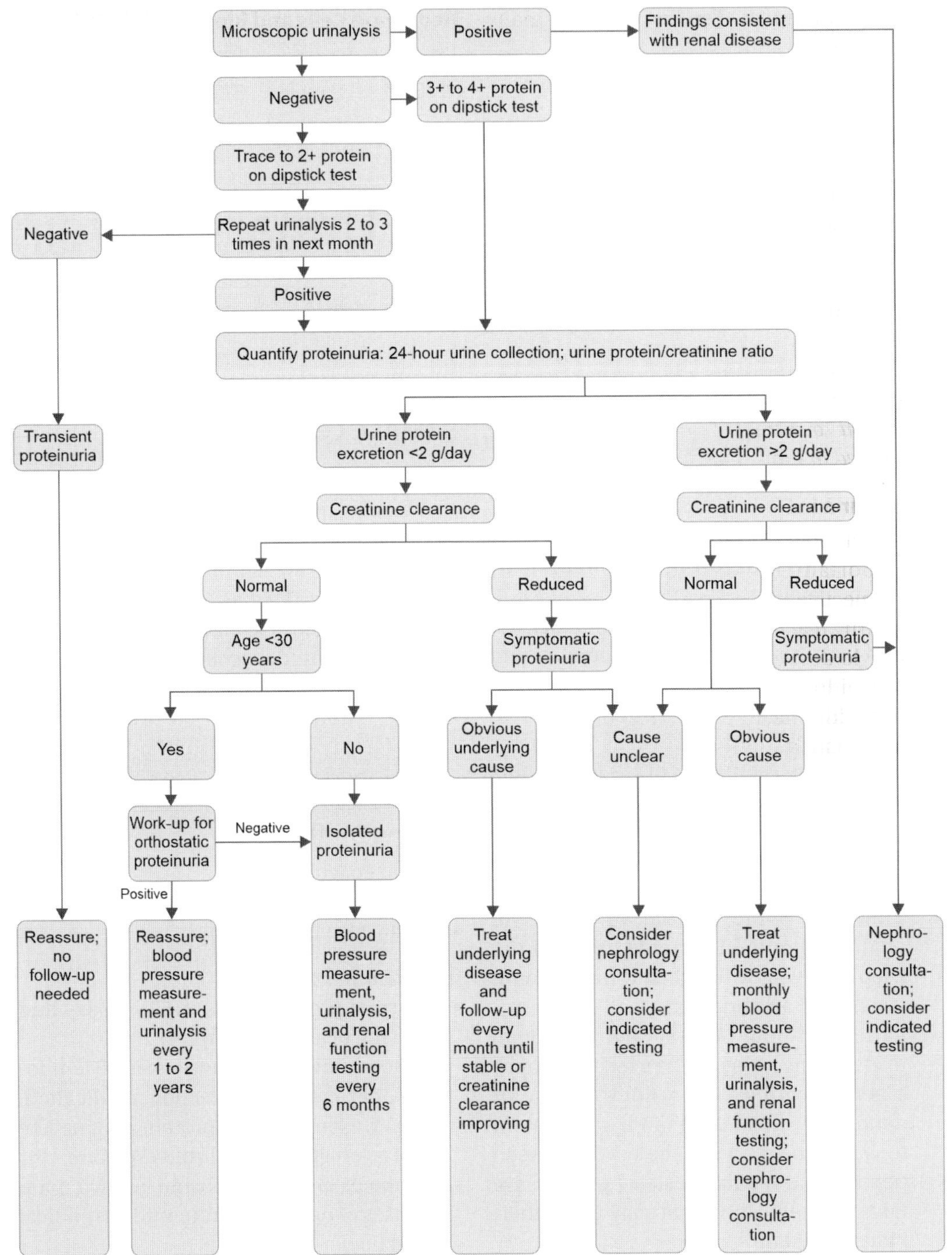

FLOWCHART 1: Approach to a case of proteinuria.

Proteinuria may also be seen with many other diseases and conditions. Some of the common causes include:

- Urinary tract infection (UTI)
- Pre-eclampsia
- Lupus
- Multiple myeloma
- Amyloidosis
- Bladder cancer
- Congestive heart failure
- Drug therapies that are potentially toxic to the kidneys
- Goodpasture syndrome
- Heavy metal poisoning.

*Approach to a case of proteinuria has been elaborated in **Flowchart 1**.*

Proteinuria in Dermatology

Common causes include:

- Important in work-up of cases with connective tissue disorders and vasculitis
- In drug reactions
- Amyloidosis
- Sarcoidosis, diabetes, and monitoring drug side effects, e.g., cyclosporin
- Malignancies

Red Blood Cells and Blood Cells in Urine

RBC may be present because of hemolysis, infection, urolithiasis, and glomerulonephritis.

These findings are abnormal, if:

- >3 RBC/HPF
- >5 white blood cell (WBC)/high-power field (HPF)
- >2 renal tubular cells/HPF
- >10 bacteria/HPF

Importance of Urinalysis in Dermatology

- Screening of UTI
- Screening of diabetes mellitus
- Pregnancy
- Monitoring of cyclophosphamide
- Connective tissue diseases
- Vasculitic disorders
- Porphyria
- To ensure compliance of drugs
- Many dermatological conditions require immunosuppressants, so urinalysis helps to detect silent proteinuria and infection.

Renal Function Tests

Rohit Batra, Ajinkya Gujrathi

INTRODUCTION

The kidneys play a vital role in the following functions:
- Excretion of waste products and toxins such as urea, creatinine and uric acid.
- Regulation of extracellular fluid volume, serum osmolarity and electrolyte concentrations.
- Production of hormones like erythropoietin, 1,25 dihydroxy vitamin D and renin.

The functional unit of the kidney is the nephron, which consists of the glomerulus, proximal tubules, distal tubules, and collecting duct. Assessment of renal function is important in the management of patients with kidney disease or pathologies affecting renal function.

According to the National Institutes of Health, the overall prevalence of chronic kidney disease (CKD) is approximately 14%.

INDICATIONS

- To assess functional capacity of kidneys
- To assess the severity and progression of renal impairment
- To assess the effectiveness of treatment and to know renal side effects

Renal function tests (RFT) need to be done—in cases of family history of kidney disease, elderly people, diabetes mellitus (DM), connective tissue/autoimmune disease, hypertension, urinary tract infection (UTI), obstructive uropathies, patient on nephrotoxic/chemotherapy drugs, etc.

Causes of Renal Disease

- *Prerenal*:
  - Any condition that results in reduced blood flow to kidneys
  - Severe blood loss
  - Hemolysis
- *Renal*:
  - Damage to renal tissue, glomerular basement membrane or tubules
  - Glomerulonephritis
  - Diabetic or hypertensive nephropathy
  - Tubular damage due to toxic substances
- *Postrenal*:
  - Obstruction to urine outflow
  - Ureteric or urethral stone
  - Prostatic cancer

Renal function tests can be divided into two categories:
1. Test for glomerular function:
   - Serum urea
   - Serum creatinine
   - Clearance tests

2. Tests for tubular function:
   - Urine concentration test
   - Dilution test
   - Para-aminohippuric acid (PAH) clearance test
   - Acidification test

Urine examination: It is important for assessing both glomerular and tubular function. It has been dealt in Chapter 5.

The following parameters are commonly included in assessing renal function (the normal values/reference range are mentioned).

- Serum urea (15–45 mg/dL)
- Serum creatinine (0.6–1.2 mg/dL)
- Serum uric acid (males 3.5–7.2 mg/dL and females 2.6–6 mg/dL)
- Total protein (6.4–8.1 g/dL)
- Serum albumin (3.2–4.6 g/dL)
- *Serum electrolytes*:
  - Sodium (Na) (136–146 mEq/L)
  - Potassium (K) (3.5–5.1 mEq/L)
  - Chlorine (Cl) (101–109 mEq/L)
  - Phosphate (2.8–4 mg/dL)
  - Calcium (8.8–10.2 mg/dL)

CLEARANCE TEST

Clearance of substance is defined as the volume of plasma that is cleared of that substance in unit time.

- Inulin clearance accurately measures glomerular filtration rate (GFR) as it is neither secreted nor absorbed by the renal tubules
- However, it is not routinely done in patients
- In clinical setting, estimated GFR (eGFR) is more commonly used; it is calculated from serum creatinine value.

$$\text{GFR (mL/min)} = \frac{\text{Urine inulin concentration} \times \text{Urine flow}}{\text{Plasma inulin concentration}}$$

ESTIMATED GLOMERULAR FILTRATION RATE

The Cockcroft–Gault formula is used routinely for estimating creatinine clearance (CrCl) as it provides a reliable approximation of residual renal function in all patients with CKD.

The formulas are as follows:

$$\text{CrCl (male)} = \frac{[(140-\text{age}) \times \text{weight in kg}]}{(\text{serum creatinine} \times 72)}$$

- However, this has been extensively modified and there are online calculators of eGFR from serum creatinine and body weight of patients.
- The eGFR is used to determine the stage of CKD.

BLOOD UREA NITROGEN

- Blood urea nitrogen (BUN) tests measure the amount of nitrogen in the blood. Urea nitrogen is a breakdown product of protein.
- However, not all elevated BUN tests are due to kidney damage. Common medications, including large doses of aspirin and some types of antibiotics, can also increase your BUN. So, it is a sensitive test but not specific.
- *A normal BUN level* is 7–20 mg/dL. A higher value could suggest several different health problems.

SERUM CREATININE

- It is the breakdown product of creatine phosphate in muscle, creatinine is filtered out and not reabsorbed in kidney.
- Normal range is 0.8–1.3 mg/dL in males and 0.6–1 mg/dL in females.
- Levels are increased in impaired kidney function, consumption of high protein diet, body builders, consumption of

anabolic steroids, crush muscle injury, burns, acromegaly, rhabdomyolysis and some drugs (probenecid, trimethoprim, amiloride etc.).

- *Low creatinine*: As such low creatinine has no value, but sometime can be seen in liver disease (because of less formation), muscle dystrophy, and pregnancy.

INDICATORS OF RENAL DISEASE IN SERUM ANALYSIS

- *Serum urea and creatinine*: They both are increased in renal disease.
- Urea increases more in glomerular disease as compared to creatinine.
  - Urea is a less reliable indicator than creatinine as it is affected by many factors such as protein intake, dehydration and muscle breakdown.
- *Serum uric acid*:
  - It may increase in CKD but not sufficient to cause gout.
  - However, raised uric acid is a bad prognostic indicator for chronic renal disease.
  - Total protein and albumin:
    - Both serum total protein and albumin are decreased in CKD due to increased proteinuria.
    - Even though proteinuria may also be seen in acute kidney disease but it usually does not alter the total protein and albumin.
  - Serum electrolytes:
    - Sodium is decreased (hyponatremia) and potassium is increased (hyperkalemia) in CKD as kidney reabsorbs sodium in exchange of potassium.
    - Chloride and phosphate are increased in CKD.
    - Calcium is decreased as vitamin D is deficient.

Changes in hemogram and urine analysis in kidney disease:

- *Hemogram*: Red blood cell (RBC) count and hemoglobin are decreased in advanced stages of kidney disease due to deficiency of erythropoietin.
- *Urine routine microscopy reveals*: Proteinuria in both acute and CKD as well as kidney infection.

Proteinuria can be of two types:
1. In the initial stages, very less amount of albumin escapes into urine; microalbuminuria (30–300 mg/day)
2. *Frank proteinuria (when it is >300 mg/ day)*:
   - Best evaluated in 24-hour urine sample.
   - In spot urine albumin/creatinine ratio is used to evaluate proteinuria.
   - Presence of RBCs may indicate glomerulonephritis, acute nephritis and kidney infection.
   - Presence of pus cells, esterase positivity and nitrites may indicate bacterial infection. Details of proteinuria has been discussed in Chapter 5 and 6.

TESTS FOR TUBULAR FUNCTION

- *Urine concentration test*:
  - In CKD, kidneys loses the ability to concentrate urine
  - Specific gravity of urine is measured
  - Low-fixed specific gravity is indicative of CKD
- *Dilution test*: After overnight water deprivation, patient is asked to take 1,200 mL of water in half an hour followed by measurement of specific gravity of urine in samples collected over next 4 hours. At least one sample should show specific gravity of 1.003 or below.
- *Para-aminohippuric acid clearance test*: PAH is unique due to complete excretion

in one passage through kidney as it is both filtered and secreted.

Therefore, clearance of PAH is a measure of renal plasma flow.

- *Acidification test*: In this the ability to acidify urine is tested after administering 0.1 g/kg ammonium chloride gelatin-coated samples.

HYPONATREMIA

- Hyponatremia is when Na^+ concentration <135 mmol/L
- Normal serum Na^+ levels are 135–145 mmol/L (135–145 mEq/L)

Severity of hyponatremia is defined as:
- <135 mmol/L mild
- <130 mmol/L moderate
- <120 mmol/L severe

Causes:
- *Hypovolemic hyponatremia* deficiency of both Na^+ and water:
  - Increased free water intake
  - Gastrointestinal (GI) loss (e.g., vomiting, diarrhea, and tube drainage)
  - Insensible loss (sweating and burns), burns, pancreatitis, and trauma.
  - Primary adrenal insufficiency
  - Salt-losing nephropathies
  - Phase of acute tubular necrosis
  - Thiazide diuretics, glycosuria, ketonuria, bicarbonaturia, cerebral salt wasting, mineralocorticoids deficiency, etc.
- *Euvolemic hyponatremia*: Secondary adrenal insufficiency due to pituitary disease; hypothyroidism and syndrome of inappropriate antidiuresis (SIAD).
- *Hypervolemic hyponatremia* is accompanied by a proportionately greater increase in total body water leading to a reduced plasma Na^+. It can be caused by congestive heart failure, cirrhosis nephrotic syndrome and renal failure.

Signs and Symptoms of Hyponatremia

They depend on onset of hyponatremia. The gradual onset may develop some tolerance, while the acute onset may be even fatal.

Symptoms include headache, nausea, vomiting, loss of appetite, fatigue, cramps, and sometimes coma. Usually neurological symptoms develop at very low levels of Na^+ and may cause increased pressure in the skull because of cerebral edema which causes hyponatremic encephalopathy.

Symptoms severity depend on how fast and how severe the drop in plasma Na^+ level has happened. A gradual drop, even to very low levels, may be tolerated well if it occurs over several days or weeks, because of neuronal adaptation. The presence of underlying neurological disease such as a seizure disorder or non-neurological metabolic abnormalities, also affects the severity of neurologic symptoms.

Treatment of Acute Symptomatic Hyponatremia

- Hypertonic 3% saline (513 mM) to acutely increase plasma Na^+ concentration by 1–2 mM/h to a total of 4–6 mM.
- The traditional approach to calculate Na^+ deficit = 0.6 × body weight × (target plasma Na^+ concentration – actual plasma Na^+ concentration), followed by a calculation of the required rate. The correction should be done slowly, fast correction may cause pontine myelinolysis which presents as paralysis, dysphagia and dysarthria.
- A widely used formula is the Adrogue-Madias formula. Change in serum Na^+ with infusing solution (mM/l/h) = [infusate (Na + K)] – serum Na/(total body water + 1).
- Plasma Na^+ concentration should be monitored every 2–4 h during treatment

in severe symptomatic hyponatremia, the rate of Na$^+$ correction should be 6–12 mEq/L/24 h and 18 mEq/L or <48 hours. A bolus of 100–150 mL of hypertonic 3% saline can be given to correct severe hyponatremia slowly.

- Chronic hypernatremia should be corrected at a rate of 0.5 mEq/L/h with a maximum change of 8–10 mEq/L/24 h.

HYPERNATREMIA

Hypernatremia is generally defined as a serum Na$^+$ level of >145 mmol/L.

Hypernatremia can be with normal volume, low volume and high volume.

Causes of:
- Normovolemic hypernatremia—fever, extreme thirst, tachypnea, diabetes insipidus, etc.
- Hypovolemic hypernatremia—sweating, vomiting, diarrhea, diuretic medication and kidney disease.
- Hypervolemic hypernatremia—hyper-aldosteronism, excessive IV 3% normal saline or sodium bicarbonate or rarely from high salt diet.

Signs and symptoms: Increased thirst, high Na$^+$ level may cause brain cell shrinkage leading to confusion, muscle twitching or spasms, seizures and coma may occur.

Treatment

Significant hypernatremia should be treated carefully with intravenous dextrose and 0.45% normal saline. Slow infusion is given to prevent rapid correction as it may cause brain edema.

HYPERKALEMIA

Normal potassium levels—3.5 and 5.0 mmol/L (3.5 and 5.0 mEq/L):

- Hypokalemia—below 3.5 mmol/L is defined as hypokalemia
- Severe hypokalemia when levels are <2.5 mmol/L
- Hyperkalemia is defined as a plasma potassium level of >5.5 mEq/L.
- Severe hyperkalemia when serum potassium levels are >6.0 mEq/L, decrease in renal excretion is the most frequent cause.
- Usually hyperkalemia remains asymptomatic. In some cases, it can cause palpitations, muscle cramps/weakness, numbness, if level is very high.
- Electrocardiograph (ECG) findings generally correlate with the potassium level.
- Potentially life-threatening arrhythmias occur without warning at almost any level of hyperkalemia. Tall and symmetrically-tented T waves in ECG.
- In patients with organic heart disease and an abnormal baseline ECG, bradycardia may be the only new ECG abnormality.

Treatment of Hyperkalemia

- Antagonizing the membrane effects of potassium with calcium—10% IV calcium gluconate, monitor cardiac functions and rhythm.
- Driving extracellular potassium into the cells—IV insulin and monitor blood glucose.
- Removing excess potassium from the body—diuretics/hemodialysis.

Pseudohyperkalemia

When potassium levels falsely elevated. This condition is usually suspected when patient is clinically well with no ECG changes. It can be due to hemolysis of blood sample, mechanical trauma during blood drawing, potassium leakage occurs out of RBC, severe exercise, and prolonged length of blood storage.

HYPOKALEMIA

Hypokalemia is defined as serum level below 3.5 mmol/L.

Symptoms of severe hypokalemia: Tiredness, leg cramps, weakness, malaise and constipation. It can also cause an abnormal heart rhythm specially bradycardia and can cause cardiac arrest.

Causes: Severe vomiting, diarrhea, drugs (specially furosemide and steroids), dialysis, diabetes insipidus, poor diet intake hyperaldosteronism and hypomagnesemia.

RENAL DISEASE AND SKIN

- Dermatologic manifestations of diseases associated with end stage renal disease diabetes mellitus—dermopathy, necrobiosis, acanthosis nigricans, Kyrle disease, connective tissue disorders; Fabry's disease—angiokeratomas; tuberous sclerosis—adenoma sebaceum, ashleaf macule, periungual fibromas and shagreen patch.
- *Uremic dermopathy*: Xerosis, pruritus, pigmentary alteration, nail changes, hair changes, acquired perforating disorder (Kyrle disease), bullous disease of dialysis, calcinosis cutis (metastatic), calciphylaxis, nephrogenic systemic fibrosis and porphyria cutanea tarda.
  - *Pigmentary changes*: Pallor—anemia, yellowish hue—carotenoids, and hyperpigmentation—because of increased melanocyte-stimulating hormone (MSH).
  - Purpura/ecchymosis/easy bruising defects in primary hemostasis such as increased vascular fragility, abnormal platelet function and use of heparin during dialysis is the main causes of bleeding in these patients.
  - *Nail changes*: Lindsay's nails (half and half nails), koilonychia, subungual hyperkeratosis, onycholysis, splinter hemorrhages and yellow nail syndrome.
  - *Hair changes*: Dry, lustreless, sparse body hair, diffuse alopecia, decreased sebum secretion and chronic telogen effluvium.
  - *Calcific uremic arteriolopathy (calciphylaxis)*: Calcification, intimal hypertrophy, thrombosis of small vessels, necrotizing and nonhealing ulcers.
  - Acquired perforating dermatosis (APD) – with papulonodular hyperkeratosis with central crust, Kyrle's disease, elastosis perforans serpiginosa, perforating folliculitis and reactive perforating collagenosis.
  - Porphyria cutanea tarda—bullae on the dorsal surfaces of the hands and feet.
  - Bullous disease of dialysis—It resembles porphyria
  - Nephrogenic fibrosing dermopathy (NFD)—painful, pruritic, erythematous, sclerotic dermal plaques present over arms and legs with sparing of the head and neck.
- Dermatologic disorders associated with renal transplantation include infections, side effects of drugs like steroids, immunosuppressants and malignancies. Skin changes in acute renal failure include edema and uremic frost.
- Uremic frost frequent in the predialysis era, the frost consists of a white or yellowish coating of urea crystals on the beard area and other parts of the face, neck, and on the trunk due to eccrine deposition of urea crystals on the skin.

KEY POINTS

- Hyponatremia is more dangerous than hypernatremia.

- Hyponatremia can be seen in Addison's disease.
- Correction of hyponatremia should be done very slowly.
- Steroid intake may cause hypernatremia and hypokalemia.
- Cyclosporine, spironolactone and diuretics cause hyperkalemia.
- In acute skin failure due to pemphigus, erythroderma or Stevens–Johnson syndrome/toxic epidermal necrosis (SJS/TEN) electrolyte imbalance has to be monitored.
- Electrolyte monitoring is required in diseases causing renal injury especially in collagen vascular disease.

Liver Function Tests

Sanjeev Gupta, Deeksha Goyal, Akriti Gakhar

INTRODUCTION

Liver is the largest organ of the body which helps in carbohydrate metabolism thus maintaining the blood sugar levels, lipid metabolism, synthesis of various proteins, metabolism of amino acids, and formation of urea. Other functions include iron storage, vitamin storage, drug metabolism, etc.

Various tests to detect proper liver functioning are:
- SGOT/SGPT (serum glutamic oxaloacetic transaminase/serum glutamate-pyruvate transaminase)
- Total protein
- A:G ratio
- Bilirubin
- Albumin
- Globulin
- Prothrombin time (PT)
- Alkaline phosphatase
- Gamma-glutamyl transferase (GGT)
- Hepatitis markers
- Ceruloplasmins
- Ferritin
- Liver biopsy

SGOT/SGPT

Serum glutamic oxaloacetic transaminase (GOT/SGOT): Aspartate transaminase (AST) or aspartate aminotransferase (also known as AspAT/ASAT/AAT) is a pyridoxal phosphate (PLP)-dependent transaminase enzyme which is an important enzyme in amino acid metabolism. It is the most commonly prescribed test for evaluation of liver dysfunction.

Aspartate transaminase (AST/SGOT): It is a PLP-dependent transaminase enzyme which is an important enzyme in amino acid metabolism. It exists in two isoenzymes.
1. Mitochondrial form (in liver)
2. Cytoplasmic form [red blood cell (RBC) and heart]

It is found in highest concentration in following organs (**Table 1**):
- In the liver
- Followed by heart
- Muscle
- Kidney
- Brain
- Pancreas
- Lungs

Such wide range of AST containing organs makes it a relatively less specific indicator of liver damage compared to alanine transaminase (ALT). Therefore, if AST is raised, it can lead to suspicion of rhabdomyolysis, myocardial infarction, and myopathies.

TABLE 1: Liver enzymes and their source.

Name of the enzyme	Present in
Aspartate aminotransferase (AST)-serum glutamate-oxaloacetate transaminase (SGOT)	Heart and skeletal muscle and liver
Alanine aminotransferase (ALT)-serum glutamate-pyruvate transaminase (SGPT)	Heart and only liver specific
Acid phosphatase (ACP)	Prostate
Gamma-glutamyl transferase (GGT)	Liver
Creatine kinase (CK)	Muscle including cardiac muscle
Lactate dehydrogenase (LDH)	Heart, liver, muscle, and RBCs
Amylase	Pancreas

(RBC: red blood cells)

Serum AST level, serum ALT level, and their ratio (AST/ALT ratio) are commonly measured clinically as biomarkers for liver health.

Alanine transaminase (ALT/SGPT) was formerly called serum glutamate-pyruvate transaminase (SGPT) or serum glutamic-pyruvic transaminase (SGPT).

Causes of elevated ALT:
- Viral hepatitis
- Diabetes
- Congestive heart failure
- Bile duct problems
- Infectious mononucleosis
- Myopathy
- Dietary choline deficiency

Elevated ALT levels due to hepatocyte damage can be distinguished from bile duct problems by measuring alkaline phosphatase.

Drugs that may elevate ALT levels:
- Zileuton
- Omega-3 acid ethyl esters (Lovaza)
- Anti-inflammatory drugs
- Antibiotics
- Cholesterol medications
- Antipsychotics such as risperidone
- Anticonvulsants
- Paracetamol (acetaminophen)

The normal levels of SGOT are 5–40 U/L and that of SGPT are 7–56 U/L.

Serum glutamic oxaloacetic transaminase is a relatively less specific indicator of liver damage compared to ALT, but SGOT levels are more increased in alcoholic liver disease than SGPT.

Levels of ALT and AST:
- *Low levels* of serum aminotransferases has been seen with patients of chronic kidney disease on hemodialysis and vitamin B6 deficiency.
- *Chronic mild elevation*: ALT>AST (<150 units/L or 5 times the normal)
  - Hepatic causes–autoimmune hepatitis, chronic viral hepatitis (B, C, D), Wilson's disease, drugs and toxins, hemochromatosis, alpha-1-antitrypsin deficiency.
  - Nonhepatic causes- Coeliac disease and thyroid dysfunction.
- *Chronic mild elevation*: AST>ALT (<150 units/L or 5 times the normal)
  - Alcoholic liver injury (AST/ALT > 2:1), cirrhosis, hypothyroidism, myopathy, heavy exercise.
- *Severe acute elevation*: ALT>AST (>1,000 units/L or >20 times the normal)
  - Hepatic cause: Acute Budd–Chiari, acute viral hepatitis, acute ischemic hepatitis, acute drug induced, hepatic artery ligation, acute bile obstruction, autoimmune hepatitis.
- *Severe acute elevation*: AST>ALT (1,000 units/L or >20–25 times the normal). Can be due to alcoholic liver injury, drugs or toxin induced, acute rhabdomyolysis.
- *Highly-elevated levels = (>20 times)*: Viral hepatitis and toxin-induced hepatic necrosis

- *Moderately-elevated levels = (3–20 times)*: Chronic hepatitis, alcoholic hepatitis, autoimmune hepatitis, and acute biliary obstruction.

Hepatotoxic drugs used in dermatology [requiring liver function test (LFT) monitoring]:

- Ketoconazole
- Fluconazole
- Tetracycline
- Erythromycin
- Trimethoprim-sulfamethoxazole
- Corticosteroids
- Interferon-alpha
- Cyclosporine
- Isotretinoin
- Methotrexate, azathioprine, etc.

BILIRUBIN

Bilirubin is produced by the normal breakdown of pigment-containing proteins, especially hemoglobin from senescent red blood cells. Bilirubin released from such sources, tightly albumin bound, is delivered to the liver, where it is efficiently extracted and conjugated by hepatic glucuronidation and sulfation (**Table 2**).

Therefore, the amount of conjugated bilirubin present in serum in healthy subjects is trivial (<10% of measured total bilirubin). Only conjugated bilirubin appears in urine (unconjugated bilirubin is albumin bound and water insoluble).

- An elevated level of conjugated serum bilirubin implies liver disease.
- The increase in unconjugated bilirubin is due to overproduction, reduced hepatic uptake of the unconjugated bilirubin, and reduced conjugation of bilirubin.

TABLE 2: Normal levels of bilirubin.	
Total bilirubin	<1.2 mg/dL
Direct bilirubin	0–0.2 mg/dL
Indirect bilirubin	0.2–0.7 mg/dL

- Clinically apparent jaundice appears when total bilirubin exceeds 2.5 mg/dL.
- Direct bilirubin is increased in obstructive jaundice.
- Indirect bilirubin is increased in hemolytic jaundice.

Jaundice can be divided as:

- *Prehepatic jaundice*: Due to increased hemolysis
  - Spherocytosis
  - Homozygous sickle cell disease
  - Thalassemia major
- *Hepatic causes*: Due to liver damage
  - Viral hepatitis
  - Alcoholic cirrhosis
  - Primary biliary cirrhosis
  - Drug-induced jaundice
  - Alcoholic hepatitis
- *Posthepatic jaundice*:
  - Due to biliary obstruction by a stone in the common bile duct
  - By carcinoma of the pancreas

Bilirubin in Neonates

The measurement of bilirubin levels in the newborns is done through the use of bilimeter or transcutaneous bilirubinometer instead of performing LFTs.

When the total serum bilirubin increases over 95th percentile for age during the first week of life for high risk babies, it is known as hyperbilirubinemia of the newborn (neonatal jaundice) and requires light therapy to reduce the amount of bilirubin in the blood.

Pathological jaundice in newborns should be suspected when:

- The serum bilirubin level rises by >5 mg/dL/day
- Serum bilirubin more than the physiological range
- Clinical jaundice >2 weeks
- And conjugated bilirubin (dark urine staining clothes)

Hemolytic jaundice is the most common cause of pathological jaundice.

Risk factors for hemolytic jaundice:
- Those babies with Rh hemolytic disease
- ABO incompatibility with the mother
- Glucose-6-phosphate dehydrogenase (G-6-PD) deficiency
- Minor blood group incompatibility (**Flowchart 1**).

Albumin

Serum albumin accounts for around 55% of plasma protein. About 10–12 g of albumin is synthesized in liver daily.

Albumin is synthesized in the liver and helps to bind water, cations, fatty acids, and bilirubin. It also plays a key role in maintaining the oncotic pressure of blood.
- Normal levels = 3.5–5.5 g/dL

Albumin levels may be low due to:
- Liver disease resulting in a decreased production of albumin (e.g., cirrhosis)
- Inflammation triggering an acute phase response which temporarily decreases the liver's production of albumin
- Excessive loss of albumin due to protein-losing enteropathies or nephrotic syndrome

Globulin

Globulins make up approximately 35% of plasma protein (typical reference range: 2–3.5 g/dL).

Globulins are involved in a range of processes including transport of ions, hormones, and lipids; acute-phase responses; and, as immunoglobulins, immune response.

If the globulins levels drop, binding to hormone is decreased and hormones free

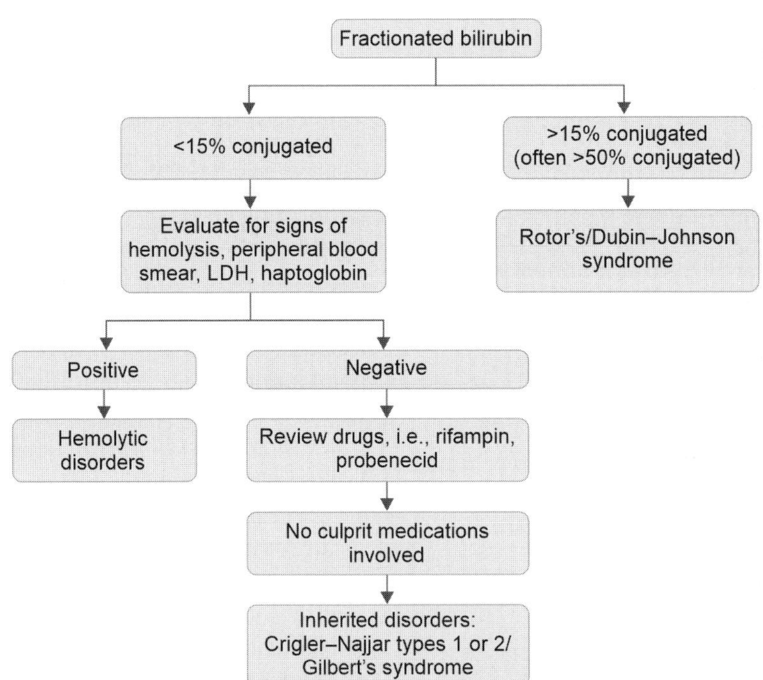

FLOWCHART 1: Approach to a case of increased bilirubin.

levels increase. Therefore, estimation of protein levels is important in endocrinology.

- *Globulins are divided into four subgroups*:
  1. Alpha1 (comprising mainly alpha1 antitrypsin)
  2. Alpha2 (including haptoglobin and ceruloplasmin)
  3. Beta (comprising transferrin and some complement components)
  4. Gamma (predominantly immuno-globulins and C-reactive protein)
- *Globulins level may be low due to*:
  - Malnutrition
  - Nephrotic syndrome when there is renal protein loss
- *Globulins level can increase due to*:
  - Dehydration
  - In response to acute infections such as pneumonia and hepatitis
  - Chronic inflammatory conditions such as rheumatoid arthritis and systemic lupus erythematosus (SLE)
  - Waldenström macroglobulinemia, a type of non-Hodgkin lymphoma in which abnormal cells synthesize large amounts of macroglobulin
  - Multiple myeloma, a malignant neoplasm of plasma cells characterized by excessive synthesis of monoclonal globulin that can usually be detected in blood and urine (**Table 3**)

Albumin:Globulin Ratio

Normally A:G ratio ranges between 1.1 and 2.5:

- A:G ratio increased in:
  - Hypothyroidism
  - High protein/high carbohydrate diet with poor nitrogen retention
  - Hypogammaglobulinemia
  - Glucocorticoid excess
- A:G ratio decreased in:
  - Liver dysfunction
  - Overproduction of globulins
  - Underproduction of albumin

TABLE 3: Different liver proteins and their interpretation.

Protein	Condition	Change
Albumin	Chronic liver disease	↓
γ-globulins	Cirrhosis	↑
α1-antitrypsin	Cirrhosis due to alpha-1 antitrypsin deficiency	↓
Ceruloplasmin	Wilsons disease	↓
α-fetoprotein	Primary hepatocellular carcinoma	greatly ↑

  - Loss of albumin due to kidney disorders
  - Paraproteinemia

PROTHROMBIN TIME

Normal PT = 11–12 seconds:

- Prothrombin time is a measure of the blood's coagulation tendency, specifically assessing the extrinsic pathway.
- In the absence of other secondary causes such as anticoagulant drug use and vitamin K deficiency, an increased PT can indicate liver disease and dysfunction. The liver is responsible for the synthesis of clotting factors, therefore hepatic pathology can impair this process resulting in an increased PT.
- Vitamin K is required for the production of prothrombin. If injection of vitamin K results in normalization of PT that means that the hepatocellular function is normal.

ALKALINE PHOSPHATASE

- Alkaline phosphatase (ALP) is an enzyme particularly found in organs like:
  - Liver,
  - Bile duct and
  - Placenta
  - Bone tissues
  - Kidney
  - Intestines

- Alkaline phosphatase is often raised in liver pathology due to increased synthesis in response to cholestasis (>4 times of normal levels). As a result, ALP is a useful indirect marker of cholestasis.
- Its levels are also increased in rickets.
- The normal range is 40–150 IU/L.
- Liver and bones are major sources of serum ALP. To distinguish between liver and bone origins of ALP, serum GGTP or 5-NT levels are done.

Physiological rise in ALP (but <4 times of upper limit of normal levels):

- Pregnancy
- Elderly (>70 rs)
- Adolescents
- After a heavy meal
- Blood group O

Leukocyte alkaline phosphatase (LAP): It is found within mature white blood cells. White blood cell levels of LAP can help in the diagnosis of certain conditions. Levels are high in polycythemia vera, primary myelofibrosis, and essential thrombocytosis.

While the levels can be low where immature leukocytes come in blood, e,g., chronic myeloid leukemia (CML) and acute myeloid leukemia (AML) (**Flowchart 2**).

GAMMA-GLUTAMYL TRANSFERASE

The GGT test is currently the most sensitive enzymatic indicator of cholestasis but it has low specificity.

Normal levels range from 8 to 40 U/L:

- Elevated levels are seen in:
  - Intra or posthepatic biliary obstruction
  - Alcoholic cirrhosis
  - Heavy drinkers
  - Drugs like phenytoin, barbiturate, abacavir
- Increased GGT and ALP activity = hepatobiliary disease
- Normal GGT activity and increased ALP activity = skeletal disease.
- GGT level has a negative predictive value of 97.9%–which is higher than that of ALT, AST, bilirubin in detecting CBD stones.

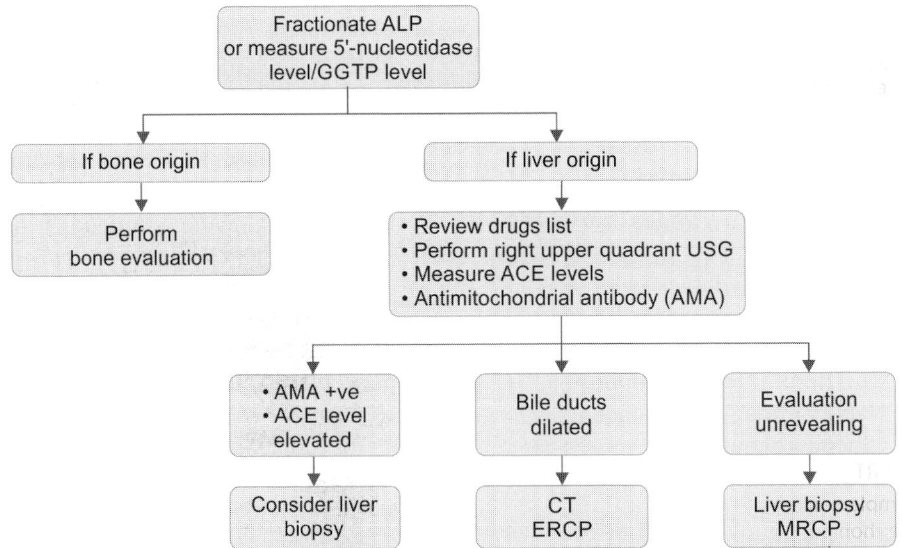

FLOWCHART 2: Approach to a case of increased serum alkaline phosphatase.

5'-NUCLEOTIDASE ENZYME

It is also elevated in obstructive jaundice, but not elevated in bone disease. The primary role of this test is to identify source of increased ALP level.

TESTS TO DETECT HEPATIC FIBROSIS

- Liver biopsy.
- *Hyaluronic acid*: Fasting level >100 mg/L has 83% sensitivity, and 78% specificity for detecting cirrohosis.

- *Fibro test*: It is also known as fibrosure. It is combination of six different test and on basis of value of these tests, score is calculated. And this score is supposed to be as accurate as liver biopsy. These tests are—hepatoglobin, bilirubin, GGTP apolipoprotein A-1, alpha 2 macro-globulin.
- *Vibration controlled transient elastography (VCTE)*: It is also known as fibroscan.
- MRI (**Flowchart 3**).

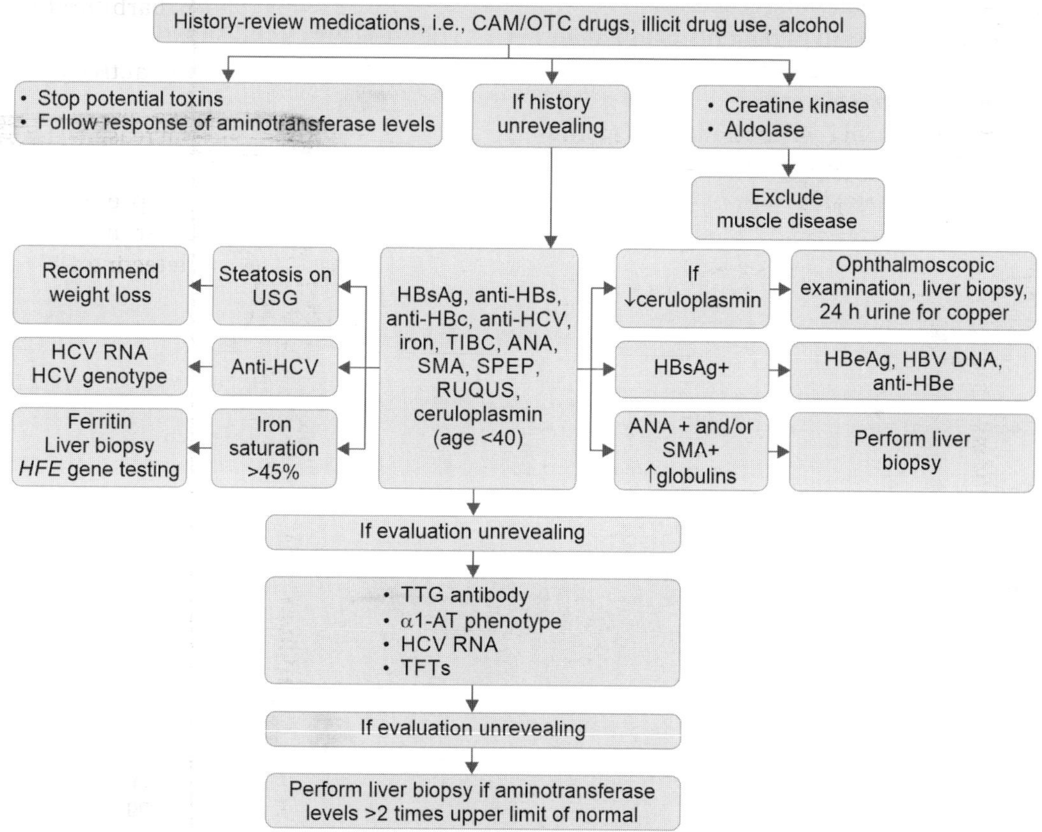

FLOWCHART 3: Approach to a case of disturbed liver function.

(CAM: complementary and alternative medicine; TIBC: total iron binding capacity; ANA: antinuclear antibody; HFE gene: homeostatic iron regulator; SMA: smooth muscle antibody; SPEP: serum protein electrophoresis; RUQUS: right upper quadrant USG; TTG: tissue transglutaminase; α1-AT: alpha-1 antitrypsin; TFT: thyroid function tests)

KEY POINTS

- Elevations in ALT generally are more specific for liver injury.
- The AST:ALT ratio can suggest a specific disease or give insight into liver disease severity.
- For complete evaluation and diagnosis, panel of liver function tests are needed. Single test fails to reach a particular diagnosis.

Importance in Dermatology

LFT's are an important battery of tests indicated in the following scenarios:

- Routine work-up of patients planned for immunosuppressives/immunomodulators, biologicals, etc.
- In monitoring of patients receiving immunosuppressives, biologicals, or any other hepatotoxic drugs.
- Patients with acute or chronic hepatitis.
- Dermatological manifestation due to liver dysfunction and deranged LFT's are as follows:
  - Spider angioma and telangiectasia
  - Palmar erythema
  - Caput medusae (dilated abdominal and chest vein)
  - Jaundice
  - Increased melanin pigmentation
  - Easy bruising, purpura
  - Nail changes like clubbing, Terry's nail, pallor, etc.
  - Associated disorders like xanthomas, porphyria cutanea tarda, vasculitis, pyoderma gangrenosum, lichen planus, etc.

Hepatitis Markers

Sunita Gupta, Amit Soni

INTRODUCTION

Hepatitis is defined as the inflammation of liver tissue.

Signs and symptoms may include nausea, vomiting, abdominal pain, diarrhea, poor appetite, asthenia and jaundice (yellowish discolouration of skin and sclera).

Hepatitis is classified as:

- *Acute*: If the period of inflammation or hepatocellular injury lasts for less than 6 months, it is characterized by normalization of the liver function tests within 6 months.

- *Chronic*: If the inflammation or hepatocellular injury persists beyond 6 months, it is known as chronic hepatitis.

Acute hepatitis can resolve on its own, progress to chronic hepatitis, or can rarely result in acute liver failure. Chronic hepatitis may progress to cirrhosis of the liver, liver failure and liver cancer.

Hepatitis is commonly caused by the viruses like hepatitis A, B, C, D, E (**Tables 1** and **2**) and rarely by Cytomegalovirus, Ebstein–Barr virus, Yellow fever virus. Other causes include heavy alcohol intake, certain

TABLE 1: Details of different types of viral hepatitis.

Hepatitis	A	B	C	D	E
Virus	HAV	HBV	HCV	HDV	HEV
Family	Picornavirus	Hepadnavirus	Flavivirus	Deltavirus	Hepevirus
Genome	ssRNA	dsDNA	ssRNA	ssRNA	ssRNA
Spread	Fecal-oral	Parenteral, sexual, and perinatal	Parenteral, sexual	Parenteral, sexual	Fecal-oral
Antigens	HAV-Ag	HbsAg, HBcAg*, and HBeAg	HCV-Ag	HDV-Ag	HEV-Ag
Antibodies	Anti-HAV	Anti-HBs, anti-HBc, and anti-HBe	Anti-HCV	Anti-HDV	Anti-HEV
Virus markers	HAV RNA	HBV DNA and DNA polymerase	HCV RNA	HDV RNA	Virus like particles

*Hepatitis B core antigen: It is not reflected in blood, it remains only in hepatocytes.

(Ag: antigen; DNA: deoxyribonucleic acid; HAV: hepatitis A virus; ssRNA: single-stranded ribonucleic acid)

medications, toxins, other infections, autoimmune diseases and non-alcoholic steatohepatitis (NASH). Most common type is viral hepatitis.

Among these hepatitis B (**Fig. 1**) and C are of more clinical significance because of high infectivity by exposure to blood, body fluids, contaminated instruments, needles, unsafe sex practices.

They cause long term hepatic and extra-hepatic sequelae.

Hepatitis A and E are transmissible by feco-oral route, subsides on its own or with symptomatic treatment and does not cause any long term sequelae.

TABLE 2: Key diagnostic points for viral hepatitis.	
HAV	• *Diagnosis*: IgM anti-HAV • Early fecal shedding-virus in stool
HEV	• IgM anti-HEV • Early fecal shedding-virus in stool
HCV	• *Acute diagnosis*: anti-HCV and HCV RNA* • *Chronic diagnosis*: anti-HCV and HCV RNA
HBV	• *Acute diagnosis*: HBsAg, IgM anti-HBc • *Chronic diagnosis*: IgG anti-HBc and HBsAg • *Markers of replication*: HBeAg and HBV DNA (mainly used in chronic hepatitis B)

*Hepatitis C virus ribonucleic acid (HCV RNA) is detectable within 2–3 weeks of exposure and anti-HCV seroconversion occurs between day 15 and month 3. Acute hepatitis C is rarely seen in clinical practice because nearly all cases are asymptomatic. So, antigen detection is not so much clinical importance.

Hepatitis-B

Viral structure consist of 3 types of antigen
1. HBsAg (surface antigen)
2. *HBeAg*: Located between icosahedral nucleocapsid core and the lipid envelope.
3. HBcAg (core antigen)

After a person is infected with hepatitis B virus (HBV), the first virologic marker detectable in serum within 1–12 weeks, usually between 8 and 12 weeks, is hepatitis B surface antigen (HBsAg). Circulating HBsAg precedes elevations of serum aminotransferase activity and clinical symptoms by 2–6 weeks and remains detectable during the entire icteric or symptomatic phase of acute Hepatitis B and beyond. The presence of HBsAg indicates that the person is infectious (**Table 3**).

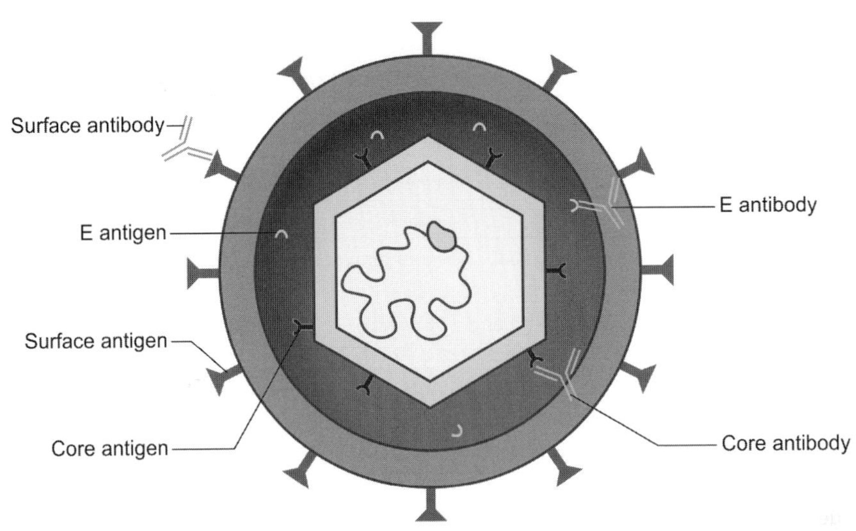

FIG. 1: Diagram of hepatitis B virion.

Because Hepatitis B e antigen (HBeAg) is invariably present during early acute Hepatitis B, HBeAg testing is indicated primarily in chronic infection, its positivity denotes active replication, hence point toward the need for antiviral treatment.

Anti-hepatitis B core (anti-HBc) is the first antibody to appear usually 4–10 weeks after appearance of HBsAg, at the same time as clinical illness and persists for years or maybe lifetime. It is almost always present during chronic HBV infection. It detects virtually all individuals who have been previously infected with HBV. Detection of anti-HBc positive donors reduces incidence of post-transmission hepatitis. It appears at the onset of symptoms in acute Hepatitis B and persists for life (**Fig. 2**).

Testing for HAV RNA/HEV RNA (hepatitis A virus/hepatitis E virus) is limited to research laboratories. HAV RNA/HEV RNA has been detected in serum, stool and liver tissue. The

HBsAg	Anti-HBs	Anti-HBc	HBeAg	Anti-HBe	Interpretation
TABLE 3: Interpretation of different serological markers of Hepatitis B.					
+	–	IgM	+	–	Acute hepatitis B and high infectivity
–	+	IgG	–	+/–	Recovery from hepatitis B
–	+	–	–	–	Immunization with HBsAg (after vaccination)
+	–	IgG	+/–	+/–	Chronic hepatitis B

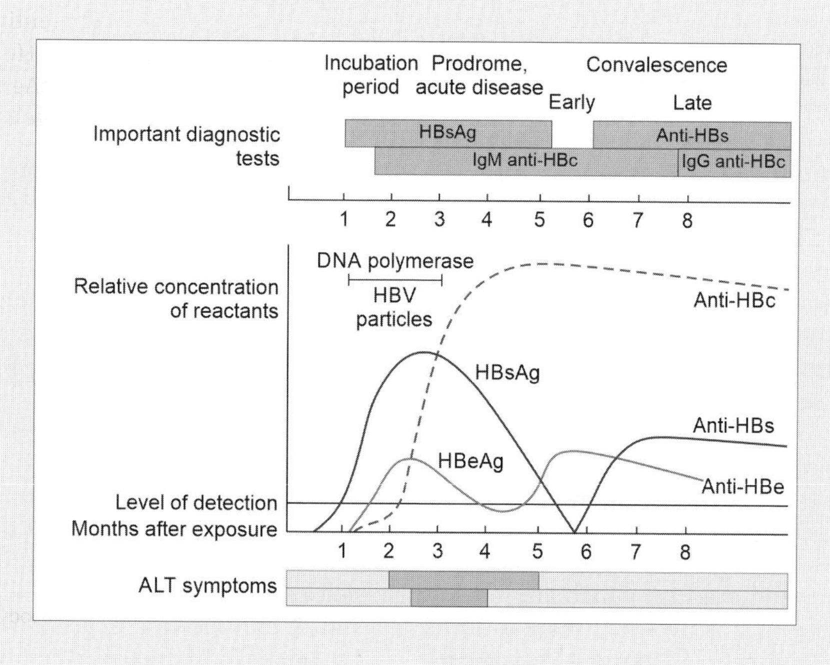

FIG. 2: Image showing titres of different serological markers of Hepatitis B and their progression over time.
(Ag: antigen; DNA: deoxyribonucleic acid; HBc: hepatitis B core; HBe: hepatitis B e; HBs: hepatitis B surface; HBV: hepatitis B virus)

antibodies of HAV and HEV appear much early, they can even be detected in preicteric phase.

Hepatitis C

It is now the most common cause of post-transfusion hepatitis in the developed countries.

Clinical Features

The incubation period is long, 15–160 days, with a mean of 50 days. The acute illness is usually mild or anicteric. Overt jaundice is seen in about 5% of patients only. The important part in Hepatitis C is the chronic illness. About 50–80% of patients progress to chronic hepatitis, some patients can develop cirrhosis and hepatocellular carcinoma.

Hepatitis C virus infection is seen only in humans. The source of infection is the large number of carriers, estimated to be about 200 million worldwide.

Mode of transmission: Infection is mainly by blood transfusion and other modes of contact with infected blood or blood products. Injectable drug abusers, transplant recipients and immunocompromised persons are at high risk. Sexual transmission is less important. Vertical transmission from mother to baby may take place.

A quarter of all chronic hepatitis cases in India are believed to be due to HCV infection.

Hepatitis C virus is a 50–60 nm virus with a linear, single-stranded RNA genome, enclosed within a core and surrounded by an envelope carrying glycoprotein spikes.

The virus shows considerable genetic and antigenic diversity. At least six different genotypes and many subtypes have been identified, indicating high mutability.

Because of this diversity there is little heterologous or even homologous post-infection immunity in Hepatitis C.

Laboratory Diagnosis

The standard method of diagnosis is antibody detection by ELISA. The third generation ELISA currently in use, employing NS-5 region protein and synthetic peptides, becomes positive only months after the infection and shows nonspecific reactions. Therefore, confirmation by immunoblot assay is recommended. In HCV infection, antibodies appear irregularly and late, limiting their diagnostic utility.

Identification of HCV RNA by PCR and branched DNA assay in blood provides more sensitive and specific results within a few days of exposure to HCV.

HCV NAAT: It is extremely useful in establishing the diagnosis of acute HCV infection, since RNA is detectable as early as 1 week after exposure and at least 4–6 weeks prior to seroconversion.

Prophylaxis

No specific active or passive immunizing agent is available.

Treatment

Hepatitis C is treated using orally administered, direct-acting antiviral (DAA) tablets. DAA tablets are the safest and most effective treatment option (clearance of infection in >90%). DAA include Sofosbuvir, Ledipasvir, Velpatasvir, Ribavirin, etc. Pangenomic drug (Sofosbuvir and Velpatasvir) combination is most commonly used for 12 weeks in India.

Causes of elevated serum aminotransferase levels:

- *Chronic, mild elevations, alanine aminotransferase/aspartate aminotransferase (>150 U/L or five times normal)*: Hepatic causes, alcohol-related liver injury, cirrhosis, chronic viral hepatitis (B, C, and D), medications/toxins, steatosis steatohepatitis and autoimmune hepatitis

- *Severe, acute elevations, ALT / AST (>1,000 U/L or 20–25 times normal)*: Acute viral hepatitis, acute Budd–Chiari syndrome, autoimmune hepatitis, ischemic hepatitis and medications/toxins.

KEY POINTS

Hepatitis B

- *HBsAg*: It is the first marker to appear in blood after infection.
- *Anti-HBs*: It the protective antibody and appears after the disappearance of HBsAg and persists in the blood for many years. The presence of IgG anti-HBs without the presence of other serological markers indicates immunity following vaccination.
- *HBcAg*: It is not detectable in blood because of it being particulate and being enclosed within the HBsAg coat.
- *Anti-HBc*: It is done only in doubtful cases to confirm acute or chronic infection with hepatitis B. It forms a clue and also excludes other causes of hepatitis such as drugs or autoimmune etiology. Presence of IgM or IgG anti-HBc indicates recent or remote infection with hepatitis B respectively.
- *HBeAg*: It provides information about relative infectivity. The disappearance of HBeAg coincides with the decrease of transaminase levels in blood.
- *Anti-HBe*: The disappearance of HBeAg in the blood is followed by the appearance of Anti-HBe. Its presence indicates low infectivity. Its testing is indicated only in carriers and chronic infection with hepatitis B. Not done routinely.
- *HBV DNA*: It is done to detect active infection and to detect the viral load and is a guide to decide the treatment protocol of hepatitis B.

Hepatitis C

- Earliest serological investigation to become positive is viral RNA detection by Nucleic acid amplification tests such as PCR (few days to week).
- It can be both qualitative and quantitative. Latter is preferred of the two, because of the increased specificity and sensitivity. Also it provides viral load assessment at the baseline, critical for determining response kinetics during therapy.

Importance in Dermatology

- Increased frequency of HBV infection is reported in telangiectasia macularis multiplex acquisita, mixed cryoglobulinemia (MC), polyarteritis nodosa (PAN), Gianotti–Crosti syndrome (GCS), chronic urticaria and porphyria cutanea tarda.
- HCV also induces extrahepatic manifestations such as MC, porphyria cutanea tarda, leukocytoclastic vasculitis, lichen planus (LP), sicca syndrome, urticaria, pruritus, thrombocytopenic purpura and psoriasis.

Lipid Profile

Sunita Gupta, Rohit Batra

INTRODUCTION

- A blood lipid profile measures the levels of each type of fat in the blood, i.e., total cholesterol, low-density lipoprotein (LDL) cholesterol, high-density lipoprotein (HDL) cholesterol and triglycerides.
- Cholesterol is one of major type of fat which is produced by the body and also comes from the diet especially animal products. Cholesterol is required in body to maintain the normal function of the cells.
- It is also a precursor of various critical substances such as adrenal and gonadal steroid hormones and bile acids.
- High level of cholesterol leads to coronary artery disease (**Table 1**).
- Blood cholesterol level is linked with dietary intake and genetic factors.
- Triglycerides are another type of fat found in the blood which is obtained from the diet and also synthesized by the liver. Triglycerides are fatty acid esters of glycerol and represent the fat depots of animals. The levels are mainly influenced by diet such as sugar, fat or alcohol but can also be high in obese, hypothyroidism, liver disease, and genetic conditions. High levels of triglycerides are related to a higher risk of heart and blood vessel disease (**Table 1**).

TABLE 1: Interpretation of cholesterol and triglyceride levels.

Total cholesterol level	Total cholesterol category
<200 mg/dL	Desirable
200–239 mg/dL	Borderline high
240 mg/dL and above	High
Triglyceride level	**Triglyceride category**
<150 mg/dL	Normal
150–199 mg/dL	Borderline high
200–499 mg/dL	High
500 mg/dL and above	Very high

- Blood lipids are insoluble in water so need to be transported by carriers in the plasma with various lipoprotein particles. Most of the circulating cholesterol is found in three major lipoprotein fractions for e.g., very low-density lipoprotein (VLDL), LDL, and HDL. Composition of different lipoproteins is shown in **Figure 1**.
- Many of the laboratories measure only three quantities namely total cholesterol, HDL, and triglycerides. From these three values, LDL and VLDL may be calculated according to Friedewald's equation:
  - LDL (in mg/dL) = Total cholesterol – HDL – TG/5
    (where TG/5 is an estimate of VLDL)

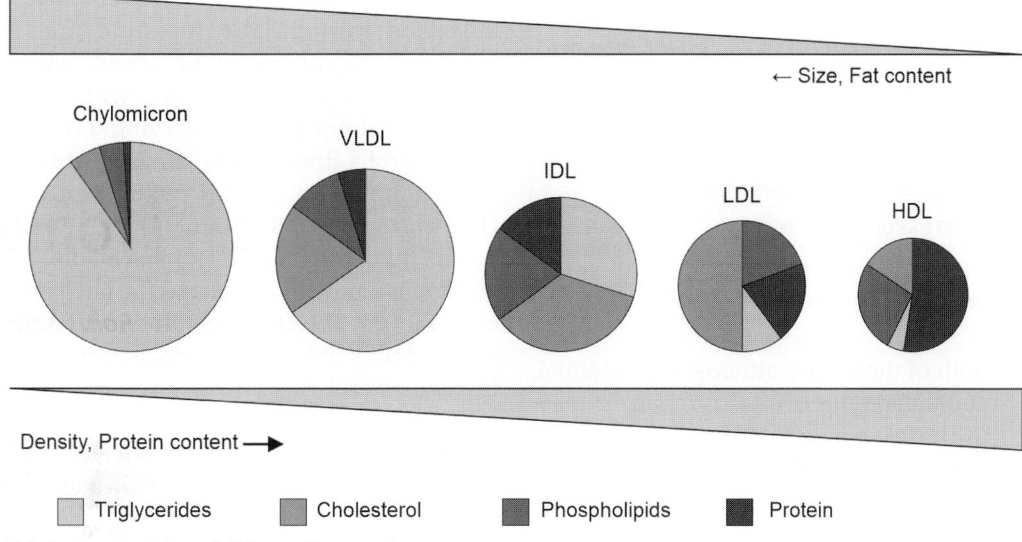

FIG. 1: Composition of different lipoproteins.

- VLDL or triglyceride levels can be calculated if we know the value of any of these.
- Triglyceride levels = VLDL × 5 or
  VLDL = triglyceride/5
- High-density lipoprotein is a biochemical combination of lipid and protein found in the blood. It is called "Good cholesterol" because it removes excess cholesterol from the blood and takes it to the liver. Benefits from raising HDL extended until the level reached 90 mg/dL, but then leveled off, which suggests no further benefits and even harmful effect may be there with higher levels. HDL can be improved by consuming a variety of fruits and vegetables and grain products, including whole grains, as well as including fat-free, low-fat dairy products, fish, legumes, poultry, lean meats and by doing regular exercise (**Table 2**).
- Low-density lipoprotein is a biochemical combination of lipid and protein. It contains more fat and less protein responsible for its low density. It is called "Bad cholesterol", as it picks up cholesterol

TABLE 2: Interpretation of HDL levels.	
High-density lipoprotein (HDL) cholesterol level	**HDL cholesterol category**
<40 mg/dL	Low (representing increased risk of heart disease)
60 mg/dL and above	High (cardioprotective)

from the blood and takes it to the other body cells. A high LDL level is related to a higher risk of heart and blood vessel disease.

To calculate LDL, Friedewald equation is used, a more expedient way to assess LDL compared with actually measuring it (which involves a cumbersome and expensive process called ultracentrifugation). It is calculated from measured values of total cholesterol, triglycerides and HDL according to the relationship as mentioned above (**Table 3**).

- Now-a-days, a new concept of non-HDL cholesterol is emerging. It is total cholesterol value minus HDL cholesterol, i.e., sum of VLDL and LDL values. As

TABLE 3: Interpretation of LDL levels.

LDL cholesterol level	LDL cholesterol category
<100 mg/dL	Optimal
100–129 mg/dL	Near optimal/above optimal
130–159 mg/dL	Borderline high
160–189 mg/dL	High
190 mg/dL and above	Very high

(LDL: low-density lipoprotein)

both of these have atherogenic potential, combined value of these gives an estimate of long-term probability of risk of cardiovascular and other diseases.

- For healthy adults with no cardiovascular risk factors, guidelines recommend screening once every 5 years for risk factors for cardiovascular disease and rarely pancreatitis.

In practice, patients are classified more broadly as having hypercholesterolemia, hypertriglyceridemia, combined (or mixed) dyslipidemia or other dyslipidemia, with further characterization and diagnosis wherever possible based on further tests.

Effect of fasting: Traditionally, most laboratories recommend 9–12 hours of fasting before screening. However, some studies have questioned the utility of fasting state before lipid panel testing. There may be false rise in triglyceride levels after meals.

Several medications have been reported to affect the lipid profile like antihypertensive drugs like thiazide, loop diuretics, β-blockers, corticosteroids, antiviral drugs, estrogen and retinoids.

Cost of lipid profile range from ₹300 to 700.

LIPID METABOLISM

Exogenous and endogenous fat-transport pathways: Dietary fat is in the form of cholesterol, triglycerides (TG), etc., which is absorbed through the intestine and is packaged to form chylomicrons, which is a complex structure coated with phospholipids, lipoproteins carrying TG, and cholesterol (since lipids are not able to circulate in blood without carrier proteins) (**Fig. 1**). In the capillaries of fat and muscle tissue, the triglyceride is cleaved by the enzyme lipoprotein lipase and the fatty acids are removed. The chylomicron remnants are released back in blood and reach liver. When the cholesterol-rich chylomicron remnants reach the liver, they bind to specialized receptors and are taken into liver cells. Their cholesterol either is secreted into the intestine (mostly as bile acids) or is packaged with triglyceride in VLDL particles and secreted into the circulation, inaugurating the endogenous pathway. Again, the triglyceride is removed in fat or muscle, leaving cholesterol-rich IDL. Some IDL binds to liver LDL receptors and is rapidly taken up by liver cells; the remainder stays in the circulation and is converted into LDL. Most of the LDL binds to receptors on liver or other cells and is removed from the circulation. Cholesterol leaching from cells binds to HDL and is esterified by the enzyme lecithin cholesterol acyltransferase (LCAT). The esters are transferred to intermediate-density lipoprotein (IDL) and then LDL and are eventually taken up again by cells.

The different lipoproteins are synthesized by liver and vary in size and density, which is inversely proportional. Meaning that HDL is of highest density but of smallest size. The triglyceride level is maximum in VLDL and lowest in HDL. The protein amount is maximum in HDL and lowest in LDL. The protein content decreases as we move from HDL-LDL-VLDL-ultra low density lipoprotein (**Fig. 2**). That is why HDL is able to remove excess fat from cells, bring it to liver as it has the highest protein content and therefore,

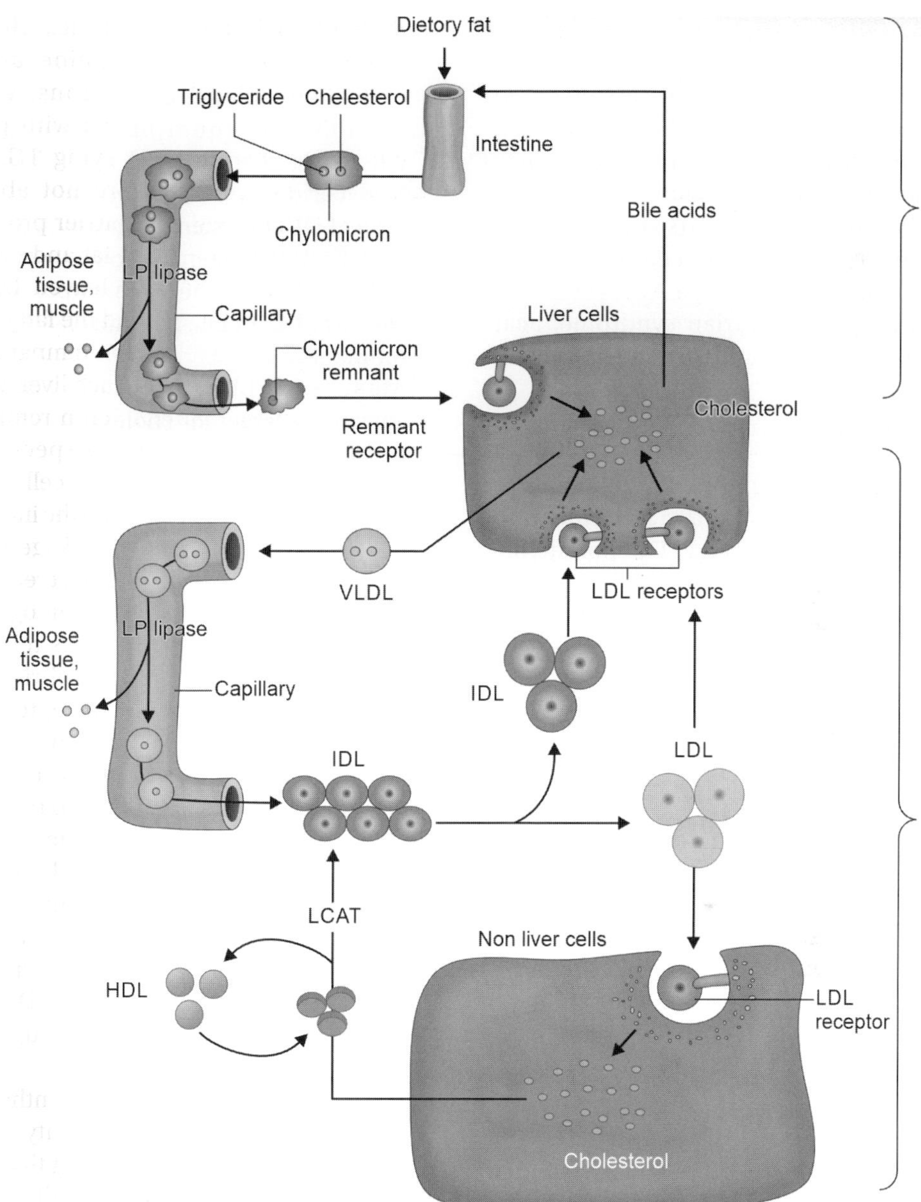

FIG. 2: Diagram showing overview of fat metabolism.

(HDL: high-density lipoprotein; IDL: intermediate-density lipoprotein; LCAT: lecithin cholesterol acyltransferase; LDL: low-density lipoprotein; VLDL: very low-density lipoprotein)

known as good cholesterol. While, the LDL transport more fat to the tissues so called bad cholesterol. This process of transportation of fat from gut- blood- cells-liver- bile-gut and then back again causes excretion of fat in some amount in stools.

Lipid profile in dermatology:
- Workup for all types of Xanthomas.
- Many dermatological diseases are associated with metabolic syndrome, e.g., psoriasis, lichen planus, androgenetic alopecia, adult acne, etc.
- Workup for patients on retinoids, estrogens, oral contraceptives, steroids, cyclosporine, etc.
- In polycystic ovarian syndrome, acanthosis nigricans and Cushing syndrome.

KEY POINTS

- Three serial samples 1 week apart are recommended for total cholesterol, triglycerides, HDL and LDL cholesterol.
- A complete lipoprotein profile is recommended as the initial test for evaluating cholesterol.
- Friedewald equation is accurate when triglyceride level is <400, when triglycerides are >400 measurement of direct LDL cholesterol is recommended.
- Non-HDL cholesterol is considered as an indicator of all atherogenic lipoproteins such as LDL, VLDL, Lpa and chylomicron remnants.
- Along with LDL, it is considered as coprimary target for cholesterol lowering therapy.

Glucose-6-phosphate Dehydrogenase

Sanjeev Gupta, Aastha Sharma

INTRODUCTION

- Glucose-6-phosphate dehydrogenase (G6PD) is an enzyme in hexose monophosphate pathway (HMP).
- It is a rate limiting enzyme in nicotinamide adenine dinucleotide phosphate (NADP/NADPH) pathway and maintain the NADPH in reduced form. This NADPH is needed for the maintenance of glutathione in reduced form which is a potent free radical scavenger and prevents oxidative damage.
- It also helps in the normal processing of carbohydrates and prevents red blood cell (RBC) damage from free radicals.
- Glucose-6-phosphate dehydrogenase level deficiency is commonly seen in males and is genetically linked, which is prevalent in African region.
- Red blood cells are mainly affected by deficiency of G6PD, resulting in premature hemolysis.
- The symptoms of G6PD deficiency may be precipitated by any infection, drug, and even with some dietary components.
- Individuals with G6PD deficiency are believed to be somewhat protected from malaria.

This condition is inherited in an X-linked recessive pattern. So, the manifestation occurs more commonly in males. This condition occurs most frequently in certain parts of Africa, Asia, the Mediterranean, and the Middle East. It affects about one in 10 African-American males in the United States.

TRIGGERS

Carriers of the underlying mutation do not show any symptoms unless their RBCs are exposed to certain triggers, which can be of four main types:

1. Foods—mainly fava beans (broad beans)—condition called favism
2. Drugs are important trigger which include primaquine, dapsone, sulfonamide, cotrimoxazole, sulfasalazine, nalidixic acid, nitrofurantoin, methyl dopa, methylene blue and fluoroquinolones. Less common drugs are chloroquine, thiazides, chloramphenicol, hydralazine, procainamide, probenecid, colchicine and vitamin C.
3. Moth balls (naphthalene)
4. Stress from a bacterial or viral infection

To prevent hemolytic anemia, G6PD carriers need to avoid abovementioned triggers.

DIAGNOSIS

Investigations are performed to get evidence of hemolysis which can occur after some trigger as explained above. Symptoms of hemolysis include shortness of breath, jaundice or yellowing of the skin and sclera dark urine, rapid heart rate, fever, fatigue, dizziness, etc.

Investigations are required to confirm hemolysis and to check G6PD level.

Markers of hemolysis in G6PD deficiency:
- Heinz bodies seen in RBCs in peripheral blood smear
- *Liver enzymes*: To exclude other causes of jaundice.
- *Lactate dehydrogenase*: Increases during hemolysis and also indicate severity of hemolysis.
- *Haptoglobin*: Decreases during intravascular hemolysis
- *Coomb's test (a direct antiglobulin test)*: Test is positive in immune-mediated hemolysis. So, in cases with G6PD deficiency it will be negative.

Glucose-6-phosphate dehydrogenase estimation is done by two methods:
1. *Qualitative test*: Beutler fluorescent spot test, rapid, inexpensive test and best for resource poor settings. On the basis of fluorescence intensity, result is classified as normal (moderate to strong fluorescence after 5 minutes and strong fluorescence after 10 minutes), intermediate (weak fluorescence after 5 minutes and weak to moderate fluorescence after 10 minutes), and deficient (very faint or no fluorescence after 10 minutes).

   Glucose-6-phosphate dehydrogenase deficiency estimation test is reported as POSITIVE, if the blood spot fails to fluoresce under ultraviolet light.

2. *Quantitative tests*: A normal or no G6PD deficiency value for adults is 5.5–20.5 units/g of hemoglobin.

   High levels of G6PD may initiate lipogenesis and adipogenesis.

The World Health Organization classifies G6PD genetic variants into five classes, the first three of which are deficiency states.
- *Class I*: Severe deficiency (<10% activity) with chronic (nonspherocytic) hemolytic anemia
- *Class II*: Severe deficiency (<10% activity) and with intermittent hemolysis
- *Class III*: Moderate deficiency (10–60% activity) and hemolysis with stressors only
- *Class IV*: Nondeficient variant and no clinical sequelae
- *Class V*: Increased enzyme activity and no clinical sequelae

Differential Diagnosis

Pyruvate kinase deficiency, which is an inherited metabolic disorder of the enzyme pyruvate kinase, which affects the survival of RBCs.

Hereditary spherocytosis, methemoglobinemia, and hemolytic disease of the newborn.

TREATMENT APPROACH

- Most of the cases do not require active treatment. Antioxidants may be helpful.
- Effort should be made to find out precipitating causes and to avoid offending drugs.
- Proper hydration is very important.
- Hemolysis once started should resolve in 1–3 weeks and later patient to be treated for anemia.

- Blood transfusion is rarely needed, proper hydration and withdrawal of precipitating factor are more than sufficient.
- Splenectomy is ineffective.

Importance in Dermatology

- G6PD test is done routinely in patients planned for dapsone therapy.
- Deficiency of G6PD was found to be related to other autoimmune diseases. (A study of vitiligo patients revealed an excess deficiency of G6PD as compared to the controls.)
- Heavy enzyme defects may cause decreased respiratory burst activity of granulocytes which may present itself as chronic granulomatous infections.

Thiopurine-S-methyltransferase

Sanjeev Gupta, Aastha Sharma, Udya Chauhan

INTRODUCTION

Thiopurine-S-methyltransferase (TPMT) is a cytosolic, methylating enzyme involved in thiopurine metabolism, located in red blood cells. It metabolizes thiopurines such as azathioprine, mercaptopurine (MP) and 6-thioguanine to inactive metabolites. In case of TPMT deficiency the inactive metabolites are not formed leading to excess of toxic metabolites.

METABOLISM OF AZATHIOPRINE

Azathioprine is an immunosuppressant that belongs to the drug class of thiopurines. It is a prodrug that is rapidly transformed in vivo into 6-MP which is further metabolized by three pathways (**Fig. 1**):

1. Methylation of 6-MP to 6-methyl-mercaptopurine (6-MMP) catalyzed by TPMT, 6-MMP is biologically inactive.
2. Oxidation of 6-MP to 6-thiouric acid, catalyzed by xanthine oxidase (XO), 6-thiouric acid is also biologically inactive.
3. Conversion of 6-MP, by a number of enzymatic steps to 6-thioguanine nucleotides (6-TGNs), which are the active metabolites.

Thiopurine-S-methyltransferase catalyzes the conversion of 6-MP to inactive 6-MMP and it also inactivates 6-thioinosine mono-phosphate (6-TIMP) and 6-thioguanine by methylation.

Thiopurine-S-methyltransferase deficiency is a genetic disorder and its activity is inherited as a codominant trait. TPMT activity varies greatly between individuals

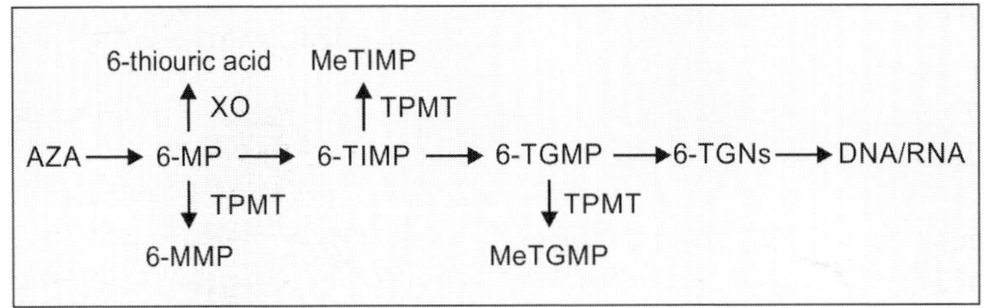

FIG. 1: Metabolism of azathioprine.

(AZA: azathioprine; MeTIMP: methyl-thioinosine monophosphate; MMP: methylmercaptopurine; MP: mercaptopurine; TGMP: tioguanine monophosphate; TGN: thioguanine nucleotide; TPMT: thiopurine S-methyltransferase; XO: xanthine oxidase)

TABLE 1: Doses of azathioprine according to levels of TPMT.

TPMT levels	Value	Therapeutic recommendations for azathioprine
High	>19	Up to 2.5 mg/kg/day
Medium	13.7–19	Up to 1.5 mg/kg/day
Low	5–13.7	Consider alternative agents or up to 0.5 mg/kg/day

because of genetic polymorphism in the *TPMT* gene ranging from normal to absent enzyme activity. In individuals with inherited TPMT deficiency, exposure to standard doses of azathioprine or MP can result in excessive production and toxic accumulation of 6-TGNs which can cause severe bone marrow suppression and consequent pancytopenia. In those with zero enzyme activity, the excessive TGN production can cause life-threatening myelosuppression (**Table 1**).

The prevalence of defective TPMT alleles varies with ethnicity. In Caucasians, approximately 10% of the population had at least one of the defective alleles. A small proportion (0.3–0.5%) of the Caucasian population is completely deficient in TPMT function. As opposed to Caucasians, Asians are much less likely to be TPMT-deficient with <5% of the population having one defective allele and almost none of them being a homozygote. Therefore, TPMT testing in Asians may not be as useful as in Caucasians.

Methods for measuring TPMT: TPMT testing—there are two different ways to assess the risk of thiopurine therapy in an individual:
- TPMT phenotypic test—this test detects the level of TPMT enzyme in red blood cells. Depending on the level of enzyme the dose may be titrated.
- TPMT genotypic test—this is an alternative test to enzymatic level estimation, this test detects the genetic variation in genes or alleles responsible for levels of TPMT.

There is diversity of genotypic variations among different ethnicities, which makes it difficult to create a genetic test to identify all possible mutations in TPMT leading to low activity phenotype.

Genotypic test can be used to interpret enzymatic levels as the number of wild type alleles are directly proportional to enzymatic activity as described below:
- Homozygous wild type—high TPMT activity
- Heterozygous wild type—medium TPMT activity
- Homozygous mutant allele—low TPMT activity.
- Measurement of erythrocyte TPMT activity
- Polymerase chain reaction (PCR) genotyping of TPMT—it is rapid

Normal range of TPMT is 9.3–17.6 units/mL (values may vary slightly from lab to lab) red blood cells (it can vary because of many physiological and some environmental factors such as recent blood transfusions, certain medications, alcohol, smoking and deranged renal function). For more reliable results we should do both, i.e., genotype and phenotype tests. However, these tests do not obviate the need for regular hematological monitoring during azathioprine therapy.

FOOD AND DRUG ADMINISTRATION RECOMMENDATION

The FDA recommends TPMT genotyping or phenotyping (by measurement of TPMT activity in erythrocytes) before starting treatment with azathioprine. This allows patients who are at increased risk for toxicity to be identified and for the starting dose of azathioprine to be reduced, or for an alternative therapy to be used.

Cost of TPMT testing in India is around ₹5,000–7,000.

Thyroid Function Tests

Sunita Gupta, Sanjeev Gupta

INTRODUCTION

Thyroid gland consists of two types of cells—follicular and parafollicular cells:

- Tri-iodothyronine (T3) and thyroxine (T4) are produced by follicular cells of the gland. Calcitonin, which helps in regulation of calcium and phosphate levels in the blood, is secreted by parafollicular C cells.
- The production of hormone by the thyroid gland is controlled by the hypothalamus which stimulates pituitary by thyroid releasing hormone (TRH) which in turn secretes thyroid stimulating hormone (TSH) and stimulates thyroid gland to release thyroxine.
- Thyroid hormones are primarily responsible for regulation of metabolism.
- The major form of thyroid hormone in the blood is thyroxine (T4), which has a longer half-life than T3. T4 to T3 ratio is approximately 14:1.
- T4 converts to more active form T3 (3–4 times > potent than T4) by deiodinases (5′-iodinase).
- Alteration in thyroid binding proteins can make huge alteration in total T3 and T4 levels, specially in case of pregnancy and in patients on steroid therapy.
- Unbound fraction, i.e., free T3 and T4 is more biologically active than total levels. So, this has more accurate clinical correlation than with total T3, T4 levels.
- A deficiency of iodine leads to decreased production of T3 and T4, resulting in enlargement of the thyroid tissue called simple goiter.

The thyroid hormones act on nearly every cell in the body to maintain:

- Basal metabolic rate
- Cell differentiation
- Regulation of protein, fat and carbohydrate metabolism
- Protein synthesis
- Long bone growth (synergy with growth hormone)
- Neural maturation

THYROID-STIMULATING HORMONE

- Serum levels of this glycoprotein hormone normally exhibit a diurnal variation with a peak shortly after midnight (2.32 mU/L, between 2 AM and 4 AM) and lowest (1.4 mU/L) in the late afternoon. At the peak of this variation, serum TSH can be double the lowest value (between 4 PM and 8 PM).
- It is the first-line thyroid function test to assess thyroid status for most clinical conditions.

- An abnormal TSH is the first abnormality to appear in a primary thyroid disease, where other thyroid tests can be normal. Using TSH as a single criterion over 95% of cases can be accurately classified with respect to their thyroid state.

T3 and T4

- Thyroid-binding proteins (thyroxine-binding globulin, transthyretin and albumin) bind almost all of the serum thyroid hormones, the minute free fraction of hormone (0.02% for T4 and 0.2% for T3) is responsible for the biological activity of thyroid hormones.
- Free hormone levels are less reliable measures of thyroid function in subclinical thyroid disease, their estimation and interpretation are difficult as compared to TSH.
- Free T4 (FT4) and free T3 (FT3) are indicated as a second-line test, used to investigate situations in which TSH abnormalities are found or where TSH measurements are known to be unreliable.

Drugs that increase FT4:
- Phenytoin
- Carbamazepine
- Furosemide
- Nonsteroidal anti-inflammatory
The indication for FT3 measurement is thyrotoxicosis of any etiology, to diagnose T3-toxicosis. Free thyroid hormone immunoassays are difficult, tedious and costly.

ANTITHYROID AUTOANTIBODIES

The most clinically relevant antithyroid autoantibodies are:
- Antithyroid peroxidase antibodies (anti-TPO antibodies, TPOAb) appear to be involved with hypothyroidism in Hashimoto's and atrophic thyroiditis.

- Thyrotropin receptor antibodies (TRAb) are heterogeneous and may either mimic the action of TSH and cause hyperthyroidism as observed in Graves disease or antagonize the action of TSH and cause hypothyroidism.
- *Thyroglobulin antibodies (TgAb):* In iodide sufficient areas, TgAb is primarily determined as an adjunct test to serum Tg measurement.

Biological reference interval (normal adults):
- *FREE T3*: 1.4–4.4 pg/mL
- *FREE T4*: 0.8–1.8 ng/dL
- *T3*: 60–175 ng/dL
- *T4*: 5.5–12.3 µg/dL
- *TSH*: 0.54–5.3 mIU/mL

Hypothyroidism

Signs and symptoms include:
- Weight gain
- Decreased appetite
- Dry skin
- Constipation
- Cold intolerance
- Puffy skin
- Hair loss
- Fatigue
- Lethargy
- Menstrual irregularity
- Blurred vision
- Depression
- Joint pain

Hyperthyroidism

Signs and symptoms include:
- Nervousness
- Anxiety
- Increased perspiration
- Heat intolerance
- Weight loss despite increase appetite
- Hyperactivity
- Tremors
- Palpitations

- Oligomenorrhea
- Systolic hypertension
- Warm, moist and smooth skin
- Lid lag, stare and muscle weakness
- Increased bowel habits
- Thyromegaly (**Table 1**)

THYROID AND SKIN

Skin in hypothyroidism becomes:
- Cool, xerotic, pale and is covered with fine scales resembling ichthyosis.
- Hypohidrosis, possibly accompanied by diminished epidermal sterol biosynthesis leads to acquired palmoplantar keratoderma.
- Carotenemia, a yellowish hue may be imparted to the skin, particularly on the palms, soles and nasolabial folds.

- Melasma, acanthosis nigricans and vitiligo vulgaris are some associations.
- Hair are dry, coarse, brittle with diffuse and partial alopecia.
- The eyebrows frequently disappear laterally called madarosis.
- Nails are thin, striated, brittle and slow growing.
- The cutaneous diseases associated with hypothyroidism include alopecia areata, chronic urticaria, vitiligo and scleroderma.

In hyperthyroidism skin becomes:
- Warm
- Moist
- Soft
- Velvety and smooth simulating the skin texture of an infant
- Thyroid antibodies also detected in cases of chronic urticaria.

TABLE 1: Interpretations of thyroid function tests.

TSH	T3	T4	Interpretation
N	↓	N	T3-elderly, associated thyroid disease
↑	N	N	Physiological or biological changes, subclinical autoimmune hypothyroid, thyroxine treatment, post-nonthyroid illness recovery
↑	↓	↓	Post-thyroidectomy, post-radioiodine, autoimmune thyroiditis, hypothyroid state of transient thyroiditis
↑/N	↑	N/↑	Anti TPO antibodies, drugs-heparin, steroids, antiepileptics, amiodarone, intermittent thyroxine overdoses
↓	↑/N	↑/N	Subclinical hyperthyroidism, thyroxin ingestion, elderly and nonthyroid illness
↓	↓	↓	Nonthyroidal illness, recent t/t for hypothyroidism, central hypothyroidism
↓	↑	↑	Transient thyroiditis, primary hyperthyroidism, multinodular goiter toxic nodule
↓/N	↑	N	Nonthyroid illness, T3 toxicosis
↑	↑	↑	Central hyperthyrodism
↓	↓	↓	Central hypothyrodism
↑	↑	N or ↓	Poor thyroxine compliance
N	↑	N	Good thyroxine compliance
N	↑	↓	Either thyroxin dose to be increased, or to look into factors causing T4 conversion to T3 (high carbohydrate diet, selenium deficiency, GIT disorders, etc.)

(N: normal)

Conditions associated with:
- *Increased TSH*:
  - Congenital hypothyroidism
  - Primary hypothyroidism
  - Thyroid stimulating hormone-secreting pituitary tumors (uncommon)
  - Pituitary resistance to thyroid hormone (uncommon)
  - Drugs such as dopamine antagonists, chlorpromazine, haloperidol, iodine-containing drug, amiodarone (amiodarone-induced hypothyroidism)

- *Decreased TSH*:
  - Hyperthyroidism
  - Pituitary (secondary) hypothyroidism (rare)
  - Drugs such as exogenous thyroxine, glucocorticoids, dopamine, levodopa (dopamine agonists), apomorphine, pyridoxine and amiodarone (early amiodarone therapy; amiodarone-induced thyrotoxicosis)

Human Immunodeficiency Virus

Sanjeev Gupta, Narinder Kaur

INTRODUCTION

A number of moral, legal, ethical and psychological issues are related to human immunodeficiency virus (HIV) testing, declaring result and dealing with positive HIV status; hence, any laboratory attempting to assess the HIV status of an individual should be conversant with these issues. Testing laboratories should ensure pre- and post-test counseling for every individual and strict confidentiality is to be maintained.

Pretest Counseling

- Human immunodeficiency virus testing for assessing the status of an individual, should always be done after the pretest counseling and after an informed consent by the client.
- Testing without informed and explicit consent has proven to be counterproductive and has driven the HIV positive individuals in isolation and away from society.
- Pre and post test counseling prepares the individual to cope with the HIV test results. It is the responsibility of all blood collection centers to ensure that pretest counseling is done before collection.

Confidentiality

- The confidentiality of HIV test results should be maintained for both positive and negative reports. This is essential for ensuring respect for the privacy, rights of an individual, to protect them from victimization, discrimination and stigmatization.
- The results should be handed over directly to the person concerned, to a person authorized by the patient or in a sealed envelope to the clinician requesting for the test.
- No results, under any circumstances, should be communicated via telephone, fax, email, etc. The records must be kept confidential.

Indications of HIV testing:
- Clinical features of HIV infection
- High-risk behavior
- Hepatitis B and C coinfection
- Partners of known HIV cases
- Blood transfusion and organ donation
- Antenatal patients
- Patients with tuberculosis, especially in young patients
- Patients with sexually transmitted diseases

- Voluntary testing choice
- Research purposes

Testing Approaches

- *Unlinked anonymous testing*: This testing approach is used for HIV surveillance purposes. All the identifiers should be removed from the specimen before sending it to the laboratory for testing, so that the test results cannot be linked to the individuals.
- *Voluntary confidential counseling and testing*: This approach is followed for the diagnosis of HIV infection in an individual. This testing is done after pretest counseling and after obtaining informed consent from the individual. The test result should be disclosed to the individual only after post-test counseling. Confidentiality needs to be maintained throughout the process.
- *Mandatory testing*: Mandatory testing is recommended in India, only for the screening of donated units of blood, blood products, semen, organs or tissues in order to prevent the transmission of HIV to the recipient.

The national HIV testing policy reiterates the following:

- No individual should be made to undergo a mandatory testing for HIV.
- No mandatory HIV testing should be imposed as a precondition for employment or for providing healthcare services and facilities.
- Any HIV testing must be accompanied by pretest, post-test counseling services and informed consent. Confidentiality of result should be maintained.

The different type of tests required in HIV infection can be broadly classified into nonspecific and specific.

The nonspecific test for HIV includes:

- *Complete blood counts*:
  - Total leukocyte count (TLC) and lymphocyte count to demonstrate thrombocytopenia or leukopenia
  - T-cell subset assay:
    - CD4 T cells/CD8 T cells absolute count and ratio (CD4:CD8 ratio is reversed)
  - Increased immunoglobulin G (IgG) and IgA
  - Lymph node biopsy
  - Hypergammaglobulinemia
    - *Neopterin* serves as a marker of cellular immune system activation and a nonspecific disease marker
    - *Beta-2 microglobulin*: Low levels indicate nonprogression of HIV
- Peripheral blood film
- Renal function tests
- Liver function tests
- Chest X-ray
- Urine examination
- Stool examination (if symptoms present)
- Syphilis serology
- Glucose-6-phosphate dehydrogenase (G6PD) levels

The above-mentioned tests are done to rule out other infections and as baseline before starting highly active antiretroviral therapy (HAART) treatment.

The different tests can be based on antibody, antigen, polymerase chain reaction (PCR), viral culture and CD4 counts.

Tests for antibodies:

- *Screening tests*:
  - Enzyme-linked immunosorbent assay (ELISA)
  - Rapid tests
- *Supplemental or confirmatory (test for antibody)*:
  - Immunofluorescent assay (IFA)

- ○ Western blot (WB)
- ○ Line immunoassay (LIA)
- ○ Radio immunoprecipitation assay (RIPA)
- *Other tests (test for antigen)*:
  - ○ p24 antigen
  - ○ Viral culture by coinfection technique
  - ○ Human immunodeficiency virus ribonucleic acid (RNA) by:
    - – Real time (RT)-PCR
    - – Branched deoxyribonucleic acid (bDNA) assay
    - – Nucleic acid sequence-based amplification (NASBA)
  - ○ Real time-PCR (for viral load)
- *Alternative to classical tests*:
  - ○ Oral fluid (saliva) HIV tests
  - ○ Urine tests

SCREENING TESTS

Enzyme-linked Immunosorbent Assay

It is the most commonly used screening test.

It has a high sensitivity, which makes it suitable for mass screening.

*Generations (**Table 1**)*:
- First generation—whole viral lysates
- Second generation—recombinant antigen
- Third generation—uses synthetic peptide
- Fourth generation—antigen + antibody (simultaneous detection of HIV antigen and antibody)—HIV duo (most common)

Earlier generation of assays can detect antibody in most individuals within 6–12 weeks after infection. The newer third generation ELISA has ability to detect p24 antigen and is positive within 3–4 weeks. The fourth-generation ELISA helps in early detection of infection. By using the p24-antigen assay, window period is shortened to 1–2 weeks.

The principles of ELISA are classified as indirect, competitive, sandwich and capture assay.

False positive results can be obtained due to:
- *Technical issues (most common)*:
  - ○ Contamination of specimen
  - ○ Mislabeling
  - ○ Improper handling
  - ○ Misinterpretation

TABLE 1: Generation of antihuman immunodeficiency virus (HIV) antibody tests.		
Generation	**Antigens/Antibodies**	**Comment/Characteristic**
First	Antigens from HIV lysates	Lack of sensitivity and specificity
Second	Recombinant proteins and/or synthetic peptides	Improved sensitivity
Third	Recombinant proteins and/or synthetic peptides in an antigen sandwich configuration	Very high sensitivity and able to detect IgM antibody in addition to IgG antibody; reduces the window period considerably. Detects HIV-1 and HIV-2 simultaneously
Fourth	Detection of both HIV antigen (p24) and both antibodies, IgG and IgM	Further reducing the window period

- *Biological causes*:
  - Participants of human immunodeficiency virus vaccination program
  - Autoimmune disease
- Hematological malignancies (plasmacytoma)
- Postvaccination including HIV vaccine
- Alcoholic hepatitis
- Chronic renal failure
- Autoimmune disorders
- Connective tissue disorders
- Acute rheumatic fever
- Multiple pregnancies
- Multiple transfusions
- Positive rapid plasma reagin test
- Technical errors, etc.

False negative results:
- Technical error (most common)
- Window period (up to 3 months)
- B-cell dysfunction
- Replacement transfusion
- Late stage disease (immune collapse)
- Immunosuppressive therapy
- Malignant disorder

Rapid Tests

- These tests yield results in <30 minutes
- The results are read by naked eye
- They are accurate and have use in wide variety of situations such as emergency room, physician's office, autopsy room and smaller blood banks.

Types:
- Dot blot assays/tridot
- Particle agglutination
- Human immunodeficiency virus spot test and Coombs test
- Fluorimetric microparticle technologies
  The "dot blot" or "immunoblot" produces a color change on a particular area (dot) due to antigen-antibody reaction.

Disadvantages:
- Subjective interpretation
- Difficult to read if the laboratorian is color blind

Advantages:
- Useful for testing pregnant women in labor who have not received any prenatal care
- Helpful in detecting HIV-2 infection which cannot be detected by ELISA

It is important to note that:
- Non-nucleoside reverse transcriptase inhibitors (NNRTIs) do not work against HIV-2.
- If an individual on antiretroviral therapy (ART) is super infected with HIV-2, CD4 count will decrease rapidly but viral load will remain undetectable (as viral load detects HIV-1).

CONFIRMATORY TESTS

Western Blot

- Works on principle of immunoblot technique
- Recommended by National acquired immunodeficiency syndrome (AIDS) Control Organization (NACO)
- It is a more specific assay
- Antibodies against various proteins are detected like:
  - Env (gp160, gp120 and gp41)
  - gag (p55, p24 and p17)
  - pol (p66, p51 and p31)
- Western blot (WB) is used only in cases of unequivocal/discordant result
- Human immunodeficiency virus-2 confirmations can be done by WB, but is not available in India (except NARI, Pune).
  In a positive sample, antigen antibody (Ag-Ab) complexes appear as distinct colored

bands on nitrocellulose strip. Colored bands appear on the strip due to binding of human IgG to viral protein.

Interpretation: World Health Organization (WHO) criteria-presence of at least two envelope bands with or without gag and pol bands.

Centers for Disease Control and Prevention (CDC) criteria—presence of any two out of four, i.e., p24, gp120, gp160 and gp41 bands.

- Negative—no bands
- Positive—various criteria
- Intermediate—bands present but does not satisfy the criteria

The most common is WHO criteria. Other antibody band tests such as IFA are seldom used.

Other Tests (Test for Antigen)

- Human immunodeficiency virus Ag detection-p24
- Human immunodeficiency virus DNA and RNA-PCR
- Human immunodeficiency virus culture

Indications:
- Acute HIV infection
- Indeterminate serology
- Neonatal infection

Disadvantages:
- Repeat tests needed for confirmation
- Expensive

None of these are superior to routine serology.

p24 Antigen

The antigen test detects HIV free antigen (p24) in the serum.

It becomes detectable after 12–26 days of infection and lasts for 3–4 weeks thereafter. This test has a low sensitivity (~30%) due to complexing of p24 antigen with antibody and is not routinely recommended.

Recently antigen dissociation assay has been developed that involves pretreatment of serum to one agent that liberate p24 antigen from immune complexes.

Since antigens appear early, it shortens window period by 1 week.

This test is useful:
- During window period
- To detect HIV infection in newborn (due to maternal antibodies) (not reliable)
- During late disease when patient is symptomatic

POLYMERASE CHAIN REACTION

Polymerase chain reaction is an extremely sensitive investigation which amplifies HIV RNA or proviral DNA to manifolds. It can amplify even a single copy of nucleic acids (RNA or DNA) leading to early detection and shortening of window period. For diagnostic purposes, qualitative PCR is used.

Three different techniques have been employed to develop commercial kits.
1. Real time-PCR
2. Nucleic acid sequence-based amplification
3. Branched-DNA assay

Role of PCR and p24 in postexposure prophylaxis (PEP): Both these tests (p24 and PCR) are extremely sensitive but costly and are not freely available, hence are not routinely advised in case of occupational exposures.

HUMAN IMMUNODEFICIENCY VIRUS DIAGNOSIS IN NEWBORNS

Diagnosis of HIV infection in newborns of HIV-infected mothers is difficult due to presence of maternal anti-HIV-antibodies. They can be present up to 18 months.

A positive DNA PCR within the first 48 hours of life indicates in-utero infection.

A negative PCR at 48 hours and positive within 1 month indicates intrapartum infection.

p24 is an inferior test as compared to HIV culture or PCR as it can give a false positive result like in case of neonates. The sensitivity of p24 increases as the age of infant increases (50–75% at 6 months of age).

In neonates, PCR can be done as early as 48 hours, 1 week, 3 months or 6 months for diagnostic purposes, confirmatory serology should be done at 18 months.

Orasure (saliva) HIV tests:
- It is a noninvasive method.
- Saliva (containing oral mucosal transudate) is collected for testing. This system obtains antibodies that are comparable to or exceed those from serum samples.
- This test first employs ELISA and then WB.

Oraquick advance rapid HIV test:
- Approved in 2004
- Provides results in 20 minutes
- The blood, plasma or oral fluid is mixed in a vial with developing solution and the results are read from a stick-like testing device.

Urine tests:
- This tests for intact IgG antibodies in urine (origin is unknown).
- This test detects HIV-1 antibodies by ELISA and WB technique.
- This test is approved by FDA but not done in routine practice.

Major disadvantage: Blood tests is required, if urine test is positive due to lack of urine-based confirmatory assay.

NUCLEIC ACID AMPLIFICATION TESTING

The routine screening tests for HIV detects the antibodies but it has been observed that there can be false negative test in the early stages or in cases of asymptomatic chronic carriers. The NAAT test overcomes these problems as it is based on principle of detection of viral genes. Even in routine screening many of the patients of HIV infection may be missed by antibody tests if done alone, so in such cases nucleic acid amplification testing (NAAT) may be of great value.

NACO Strategies for HIV Testing

The first screening test has the highest sensitivity while the second and third tests are with the highest specificity. If the test gives nonreactive result, the sample is considered negative.

A1, A2, and A3 represent serological tests with different principle/antigens.

Each sample should be collected after 2 weeks of the first specimen. If the confirmatory test fails to detect by serology (indeterminate), test should be repeated at 4 weeks, 3 months, 6 months and 12 months. If test is still indeterminate after 12 months, it should be considered negative.

Strategy 1:
- For transfusion/transplant
- One test required

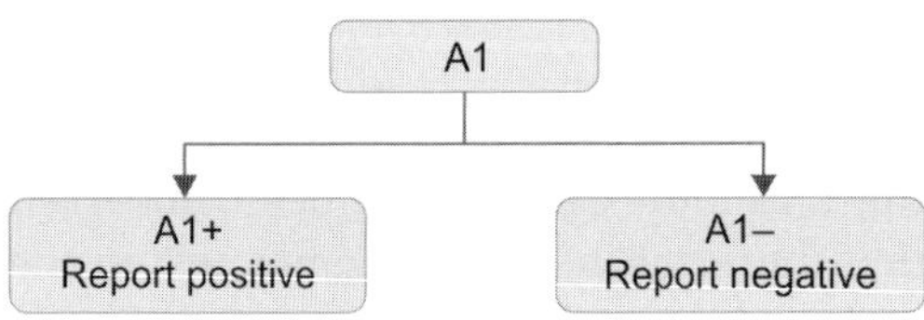

Strategy 2A:
- Used for surveillance
- Two test kits are required

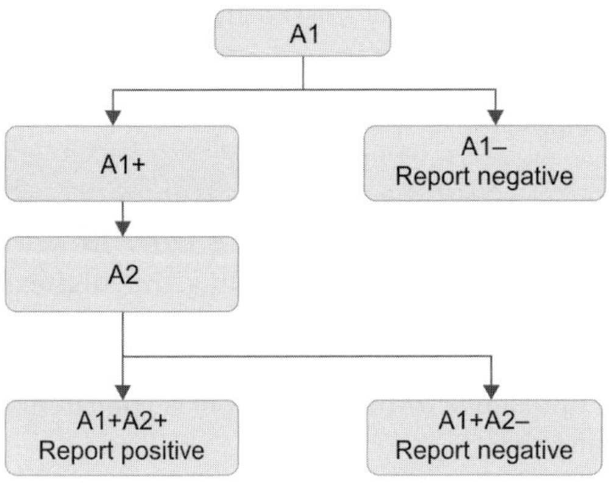

Strategy 2B:
- For patients with symptoms of AIDS
- Two to three tests required

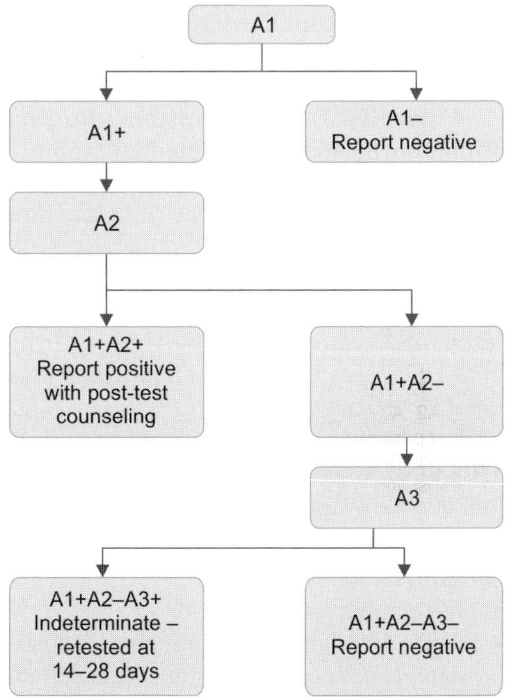

Strategy 3:
- To detect in asymptomatic individuals [in Integrated Counselling and Testing Centre (ICTC) and Prevention of Parent To Child Transmission (PPTCT)]
- Three test kits are required

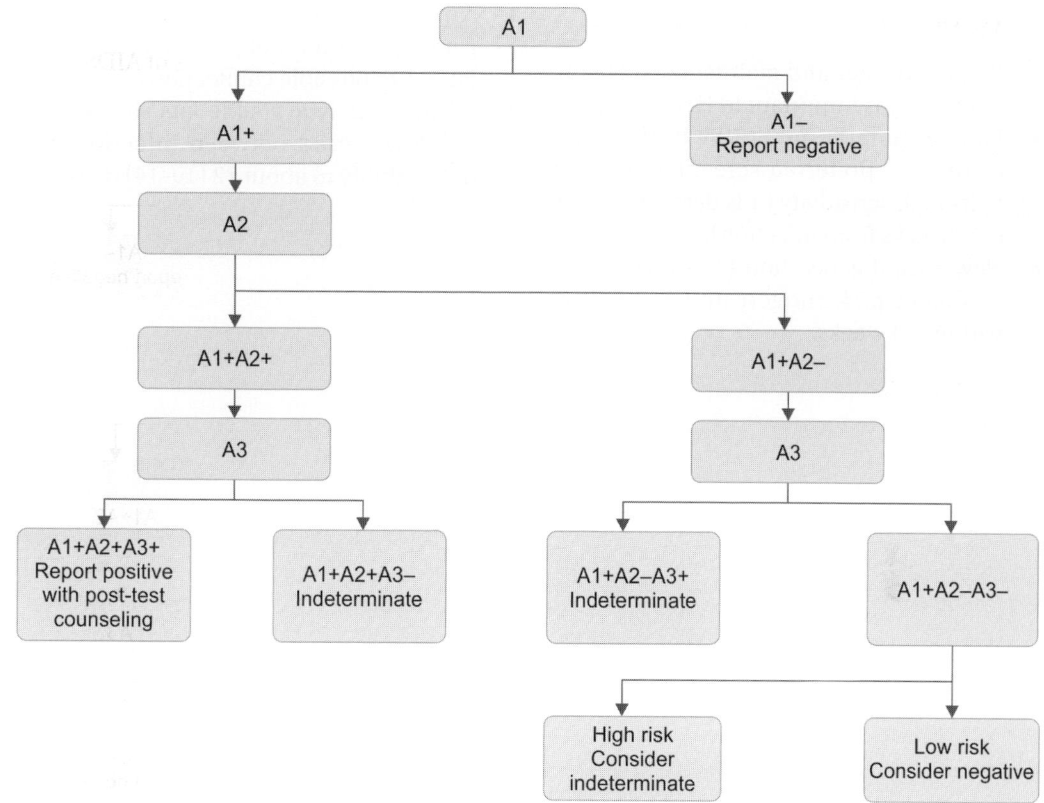

- Assays A1, A2, and A3 represent three different tests based on different principles or different antigenic compositions.
- Assay A1 should be of high sensitivity, whereas A2 and A3 should be of high specificity.
- A2 and A3 should also be able to differentiate between HIV 1 and 2 infection.
- Such a result is not adequate for diagnostic purposes: Use strategies 2B or 3.
- Whatever the final diagnosis, donations, which were initially reactive should not be used for transfusions or transplants. Refer to integrated counseling and testing centers (ICTC) after informed consent for confirmation of HIV status.
- Testing should be repeated on a second specimen taken after 14–28 days. In case the serological results continue to be indeterminate, then the specimen is to be subjected to a WB/PCR, if facilities are available or refer to the National Reference Laboratory (NRL) for further testing.

KEY POINTS

- Proper consent and maintenance of confidentiality is important in HIV testing.
- Fourth generation ELISA is the most commonly preferred screening test due to its high sensitivity (it is detectable after 6–12 weeks from infection).
- Newer third generation ELISA has ability to detect p24 antigen and is positive within 3–4 weeks.
- Nonspecific tests are used to assess general condition of patients and to rule out other possible coinfections.
- Commercially available kits shorten the window period between infection and detectability to about 12 (10–14) days.

Venereal Disease Research Laboratory

Rohit Singla, Narinder Kaur

INTRODUCTION

Syphilis is a sexually transmitted disease caused by *Treponema pallidum* which is a motile spiral-shaped gram-negative bacteria having a characteristic corkscrew motility. The organism is unable to survive outside the animal host and cannot be cultured in vitro. Its size is approximately 10–14 μm in length and 0.1–0.2 μm in diameter with 10 regular spirals at interval of about 1 μm.

Diagnosis of Syphilis

Syphilis can be diagnosed by:
- Direct detection of *T. Pallidum*
- Serological tests

Direct detection of *T. Pallidum* includes:
- Animal inoculation
- Dark field microscopy
- Direct fluorescent antibody test
- Direct tests for *T. pallidum* in tissue sections
- Nucleic acid amplification test

Serological tests for syphilis include:
- Nontreponemal tests (NTTs) or standard tests for syphilis (STS) (which are sensitive but nonspecific)
- Treponemal tests (specific)

Nontreponemal test/STS is further classified as:
- Microscopic NTTs [venereal disease research laboratory (VDRL) test and unheated serum reagin (USR)]
- Macroscopic NTTs [rapid plasma reagin (RPR) and toluidine red unheated serum test (TRUST)]

Treponemal tests further include:
- Fluorescent treponemal antibody absorption test (FTA-ABS)
- Fluorescent treponemal antibody-ABS double-staining test
- *Treponema pallidum* particle agglutination test (TP-PA)
- Western blots
- Enzyme immunoassays (EIAs)/rapid tests
- *Treponema pallidum* hemagglutination assay (TPHA)
- *Treponema pallidum* immobilization assay (TPI)

Animal Inoculation

It is the oldest and most sensitive method for detecting infectious treponemes and is used as the gold standard for measuring the sensitivity of methods such as the PCR. Rabbit is the most commonly used animal for the inoculation. The specimen can be injected intratesticular or intradermally and the material should be collected within an hour after injecting or it should be frozen immediately after collection.

Dark Field Microscopy

Treponema pallidum can be easily demonstrated by this method (**Fig. 1**). Detailed description is given in Chapter 1. This test is useful in primary, secondary, congenital, early relapsing syphilis. The sample can be collected from the lesions such as chancre and condyloma lata as well as mucosal lesions. Once collected, the sample should be immediately examined as the motility of treponemes decreases rapidly (**Figs. 2** and **3**).

Direct Fluorescent Antibody T. pallidum

This test is a modification of dark field microscopy. Sample is collected in a similar fashion, then slide is dried and fixed with methanol or acetone. Fluorescein labelled anti *T. pallidum* globulin is used to stain the

smear before examining it under fluorescent microscope. The main advantage of this test is that there is no need to examine the slide immediately. The only disadvantage is that the subspecies of treponemes cannot be differentiated with this method.

Tissue Sections/Biopsy in Syphilis

In primary syphilis, perivascular and perijunctional infiltrates of lymphocytes, plasma cells and macrophages are seen along with capillary endothelial proliferation and subsequent obliteration of small blood vessels.

Infiltrate tends to decrease in secondary syphilis. Histiocytes are present in infiltrate along with plasma cells and lymphocytes.

Polymerase Chain Reaction

Polymerase chain reaction test uses the deoxyribonucleic acid (DNA) sequences which are specific for *T. pallidum*. This test is

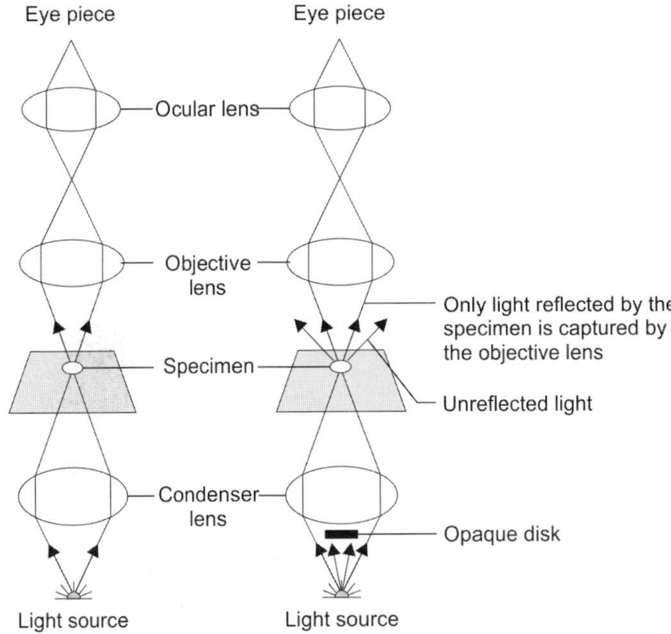

FIG. 1: Comparison of light pathways of bright field and dark field microscope.

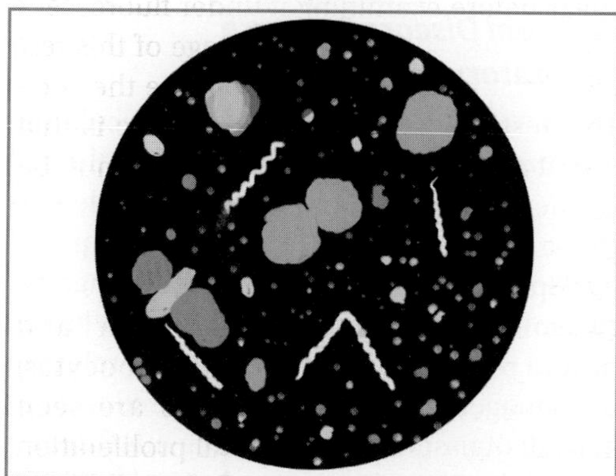

FIG. 2: Treponemes in dark field microscopy.

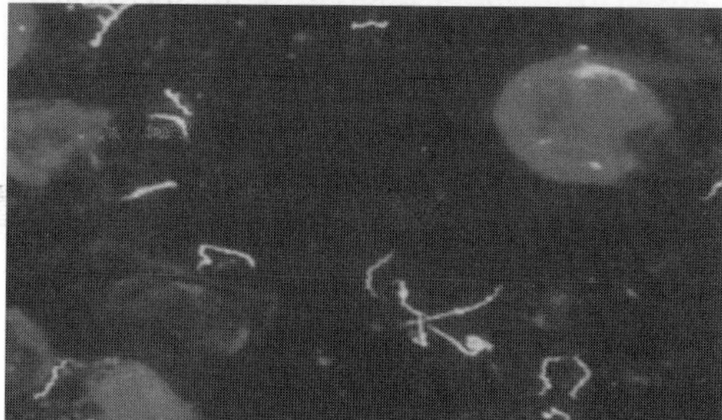

FIG. 3: Dark field microscopy showing treponemes.

specific for syphilis and can detect even few number of organisms in specimen. It is useful in early lesions of syphilis.

Serological Tests

Before understanding serological tests, it is necessary to know about our immune response to treponemes.

After nearly 2 weeks of exposure, there is formation of immunoglobulin M (IgM) antibodies (Ab) in our body and later IgG antibodies can be detected in the serum after 2 weeks. There are 20 different antigens (Ag) of treponemes against which antibodies are produced (**Fig. 4**).

There are two types of antibodies:

1. *Nonspecific antibodies*: Lipoidal antigens of *T. pallidum* are the reason for production of nonspecific antibodies in our body. These are also known as reagins. Reagins are also directed against nuclear membrane and mitochondria of our cells.

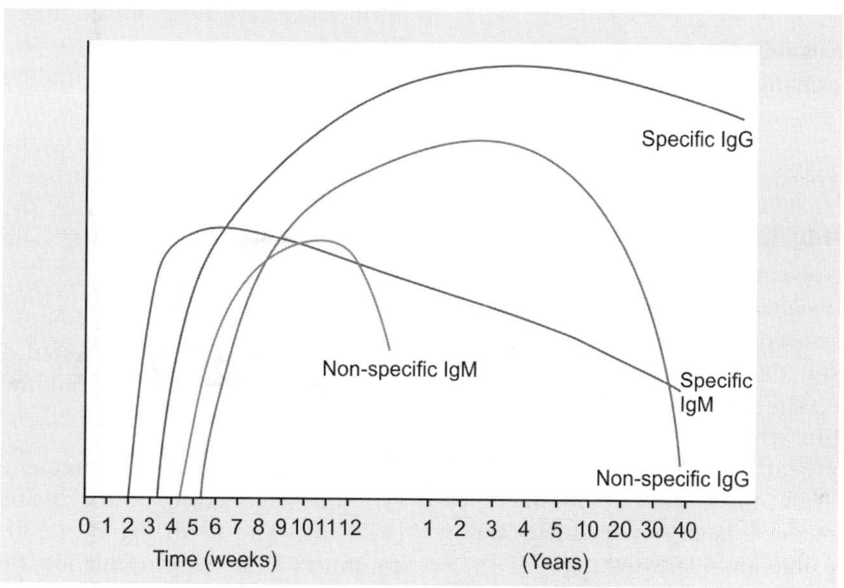

FIG. 4: Variation in the levels of antibodies with respect to duration of the disease.

2. *Specific antibodies*: These antibodies are specific for *T. pallidum*. TpN47, TpN15, and TpN17 are some of the antigens against which specific antibodies are produced.

Immunoglobulin G3 specific antibodies increase substantially in secondary syphilis. In early latent, both IgM and IgG are present whereas concentration of antibodies decrease in late latent syphilis. There is a rapid decrease in IgM antibodies after initiating the treatment. Within 6–12 months, these become undetectable whereas IgG remain for years even after treatment.

Nontreponemal Tests

All these tests measure anti-lipoidal IgM and IgG antibodies. These tests are used for initial screening and for follow-up after treatment. Except for VDRL and RPR tests, most lipoidal antigen tests are not of use now.

Cardiolipin, cholesterol and lecithin are the antigens used in NTTs. The course of the disease can be monitored with titers of NTTs. These test carry less significance in primary syphilis and late latent syphilis.

There are mainly three types of NTTs:
1. Wasserman reaction
2. Venereal disease research laboratory test
3. Rapid plasma reagin test

Wasserman Reaction or Test

This test was developed by Wasserman. It was the first test for syphilis in which the blood was used for the diagnosis of syphilis. It is based on the complement fixation principle. The antigen used in this test is cardiolipin which is taken from bovine muscle or heart. This test was later modified by Kahn. Now, these tests are not in clinical use as they have been replaced with newer NTTs, e.g., RPR and VDRL tests.

Venereal Disease Research Laboratory Test

This test is an example of slide flocculation test. It not only detects the lipid from the cell surfaces of the treponeme but also detects the antibodies—IgG and IgM antiphospholipid antibody (APA). Antibodies against cardiolipin antigen which are formed by the host in response to lipoidal material released by damaged host cells early in infection or as a result of tissue injury following infection.

The basic antigen formula used in VDRL test contains 0.03% cardiolipin (a lipoidal extract from beef heart), 0.9% cholesterol, and 0.21% lecithin to produce standard reactivity. The seroconversion occurs from 21 days of exposure till about up to 6 weeks after infection. The VDRL usually becomes reactive within the first 4 weeks after infection, peaks during the first year and then slowly declines. That is why, low titers (levels) are seen in the late syphilis. In 25% of the cases, it can revert to negative in the absence of treatment.

Antibodies reacting with cardiolipin antibodies have been traditionally termed "reagin".

- Now a days, VDRL is an outdated test, it has been replaced by RPR test because of various issues such as availability of antigen, cumbersome procedure and lack of standardization. A true VDRL testing has merely historical value now.

Procedure: The antigen for VDRL should always be prepared fresh before testing. The serum which has to be tested should be inactivated first by keeping it in hot water at 56°C for half an hour.

Qualitative test: The freshly prepared antigen (1/60th mL) is added to inactivated serum (0.05 mL) and centrifuged at 180 rpm for 4 minutes. If there is flocculation, then result is considered positive. The positive samples are then further tested quantitatively.

Quantitative test: If the qualitative test is reactive, then the titer has to be checked. Moreover, testing should always be done in dilution because the high Ag or high Ab in sera can alter the result. So, the quantitative test is performed to determine the antibody titers. Serum is doubly diluted in saline from 1:2 to 1:256 or more. The titer with the highest dilution giving a reactive (not weakly reactive) result is reported in quantitative test. It can be used to follow the course of illness, including the response to therapy.

Reporting of Results

The result of the test is defined as follows: Reactive, weakly reactive and nonreactive.

Weakly reactive can be false positive. Nonreactive means either there is no infection or treatment is efficient, but it cannot rule out infection if done during incubation period. Fourfold rise in titer could be due to reinfection, active disease or if treatment is not efficient. On the other hand, fourfold decline means that treatment is effective. After starting the adequate treatment, if titer does not decline even in 6 months or it does not decrease fourfold in 1 year, it is classified as seroresistant or serofastness.

When the test should be repeated?
- Patients with early syphilis who have been treated with appropriate doses and preparations of benzathine penicillin should be evaluated clinically and serologically (using a NTT) after 3 months to assess the results of therapy.
- A second evaluation should be performed after 6 months and if indicated by the results at this point, it should be repeated again after 12 months to reassess the condition of the patient and detect the possible reinfection.

Advantages
- Inexpensive and simple
- Suitable for mass screening
- The baseline titer can be used to follow-up the treatment response

Limitations
- Reduced sensitivity in primary syphilis and late latent syphilis
- *False-positive results*:
  - Due to technical error and variations in normal population
  - Due to antiphospholipid autoantibodies (biologic false positivity)
  - Acute false positive reaction <6 months
    - Viral infections
    - Malaria
    - Immunizations
    - Pregnancy
    - Laboratory errors
  - Chronic false positive reaction >6 months
    - Connective tissue diseases
    - IV drug abusers
    - Narcotic addiction
    - Aging
    - Leprosy and malignancy
  - Cut off value of VDRL titer for labeling a false positive result is <1:8
- *False-negative results*: If the antigen and antibodies are in equal quantities, they form flocculation, making the test positive. This zone of equivalence is defined as optimal ratio. If the antibodies are in higher concentration, the result of the test comes negative. This false negative result due to higher concentration of antibodies in undiluted serum is called

prozone phenomenon. These samples when diluted give a positive result when antibodies and antigen come in optimal ratio.

It is clinically significant in certain populations at risk like:

- Those who are on continuous immuno-suppressive drugs.
- Those who are human immunodeficiency virus (HIV) seropositive.

Also note: Antigen excess can also result in false-negative result which is known as POSTZONE phenomenon.

Variants of Venereal Disease Research Laboratory Test

Other VDRL variant tests which are not in much use now are:

- Unheated serum reagin test
- Toluidine red unheated serum test
- Automated reagin test
- Reagin screen test

Unheated Serum Reagin Test

Unheated serum reagin antigen is VDRL antigen which is further stabilized by the addition of EDTA. Therefore, need for daily preparation of an antigen suspension is eliminated. Choline chloride is added to eliminate the need to inactivate the serum by heating. Addition of choline chloride also enhances the reactivity of the antigen. USR test is performed and reported in a manner similar to the VDRL slide test on serum.

Rapid Plasma Reagin and Toluidine Red Unheated Serum Test

Both tests are based on USR antigen. TRUST and RPR card test antigens differ only in the visualization agent added to the antigen. For the RPR card test, charcoal particles are added to the antigen whereas for the TRUST, paint pigment particles are added. Particles of both tests become entrapped in antigen-antibody lattice formed with a reactive serum.

Slides are read macroscopically to determine the presence of clumping (flocculation). Results of card tests are reported as either reactive or nonreactive regardless of the size of the clumps.

All serum samples exhibiting any degree of reactivity or roughness should be quantitated to an endpoint titer.

Rapid Plasma Reagin Test

As described above, it is a card test which can give result within 5 minutes. It also uses the same Ag-cardiolipin.

Treponemal Tests

These are the specific tests where antigen is either a fragment of *T. pallidum* or the entire organism. These become positive before VDRL test but remain positive even after adequate treatment for years. These are costlier than NTTs.

Treponema pallidum Immobilization Test

This test uses the virulent *T. pallidum* (Nichols strain) obtained from the rabbits. It detects the antibody which inhibits the normal movements of *T. pallidum* in the presence of complement (specific treponemal immobilizing antibody). The reaction of treponemes in the presence of patient's serum is observed by dark field microscopy. The test is considered positive if 50% or more of the treponemes are immobilized. It becomes positive after few days to a week later as compared to VDRL test. Its specificity is 100%, but as the test is time consuming, expensive and hazardous, it is not performed nowadays.

Currently used treponemal tests are as follows:

Treponema pallidum Hemagglutination Assay

It is a microhemagglutination assay for IgM and IgG antibodies in which sensitized sheep erythrocytes are coated with *T. pallidum* (Nichols strain). The results are reported as reactive if agglutination occurs in a dilution of 1:80 or more. Reactivity can be expected around the 4th–5th week of infection. It is more sensitive and specific than VDRL as well as FTA-ABS test, except in primary syphilis.

Fluorescent Treponemal Antibody Absorption Test

It is an indirect immunofluorescence antibody test. The presence of antibody in the patient's serum is indicated by fluorescence. Intensity of fluorescence is reported as nonreactive, borderline or reactive. The reactivity begins in the third week of infection. It is the most sensitive serological test in the early stage of syphilis.

Fluorescent Treponemal Antibody Absorption Double-staining Test

In this test, a fluorochrome-labeled counter-stain for *T. pallidum* and antihuman IgG conjugate labeled with tetramethylrhodamine isothiocyanate is used to detect the antibody in patient's serum. False positivity can occur in 1% of sera.

Treponemal Enzyme Immunoassay

In this test, the antigen is fixed to the wells in microtiter plates and then serum is added and rinsed off after 30–60 minutes. Antibody to *T. pallidum* binds to the antigen and reacts in the second incubation with an enzyme labeled antihuman globulin. The result is available in 3–4 hours.

Advantages:
- Automated (or semiautomated) processing
- Objective reading of results
- Interfacing with the laboratory computer system to allow electronic report generation

Note: New algorithm suggests screening with treponemal enzyme immunoassay alone followed by an NTT.

Western Blot Technique

This technique is based on the whole *T. pallidum* lysate antigen. The presence of antibodies to the immune determinants with molecular weights 15.5, 17, 44.5, and 47 kDa appears to be diagnostic for acquired syphilis.

When an IgM-specific conjugate is used, this test has value in the diagnosis of congenital syphilis.

Limitations of treponemal tests:
- Treponemal tests may remain reactive for years with or without treatment and treponemal test antibody titers correlate poorly with the disease activity. Therefore, treponemal tests should not be used to evaluate response to therapy, relapse or reinfection in previously treated patients.
- Treponemal tests do not differentiate venereal syphilis from endemic syphilis (yaws and pinta).

Sensitivity and Specificity of Commonly Used Serologic Tests

- *Sensitivity*: It is defined as the proportion of people who test positive for the disease among those who have the disease.

- *Specificity*: It is defined as the proportion of healthy patients known not to have the disease who will test negative for it.

OTHER TESTS

- *Oral fluid test*: It is a time-resolved fluorescence immunoassay which is used to detect the antibodies to *T. pallidum* recombinant antigens in the oral fluid specimens. The specimen should be collected using "Oracol" swabs. It is potentially useful when collection of blood is not practicable. In early syphilis, its sensitivity is 100% and specificity is 97.9%. In patients with positive syphilis serology, its sensitivity is 76.5% and specificity is 96.9%.
- *Cerebrospinal fluid (CSF) examination*: It is indicated if the patient has one of the following:
  - Neurological, ophthalmic or auditory signs and symptoms
  - Other clinical evidence of active infection—aortitis, gumma or iritis
  - Treatment failure
  - Human immunodeficiency virus infection
  - A nontreponemal serum titer of >32 if the duration of syphilis is over 1 year
  - A nonpenicillin-based treatment regimen is planned
  - All infants suspected of prenatal syphilis

The typical CSF findings of neurosyphilis are:
- Moderate mononuclear pleocytosis (10–400 cells/mL)
- Elevated total protein (0.46–2.0 g/L)
- Positive CSF VDRL criteria

Also note that:
- The CSF VDRL test is highly specific and false-positive results are rare in the absence of blood contamination

- Most venereologists consider an examination of CSF unnecessary in early syphilis and prefer to examine CSF after 1–2 years of post-treatment follow-up
- In untreated asymptomatic late syphilis, a CSF examination should always be done
- A normal CSF is by definition an essential prerequisite for a diagnosis of latent syphilis

TESTING POLICY

- As NTTs are cheaper and can detect almost all the cases of early syphilis, these are done primarily when syphilis is suspected.
- When the result of NTTs come positive, confirmation is done by specific tests.
- Response to treatment can be checked with quantitative nonspecific tests.
- Every patient with reactive RPR should be started with treatment, if confirmatory tests are not available.
- There is an algorithm for evaluation of patients with syphilis, proposed by the Centers for Disease Control and Prevention (CDC). It suggests that if an untreated patient has nonreactive RPR but two different positive specific tests, he should be given treatment.

KEY POINTS

- Venereal Disease Research Laboratory is most sensitive test but not specific.
- A true VDRL is outdated, most of laboratories now shifted to RPR.
- In a clinically-suspected syphilis with VDRL negative, the sample should be retested with serum dilution to rule out prozone phenomenon.
- Specific tests are more reliable, but costly and not freely available.
- Fluorescent treponemal antibody absorption test is the earliest to become positive.

- Specific tests TPI, TPHA, FTA-ABS may remain positive throughout life, so called scar in the blood.

Importance in dermatology:
- For screening of suspected patients with syphilis.
- Syphilitic patients can present with any number of mucocutaneous manifestations. The most common symptoms were as follows-skin rash, lymphadenopathy, persistent chancre, nodular syphilides, lues maligna, patches in the oral mucosa, condylomata lata, split papules, etc.
- VDRL is included in routine battery of tests as secondary syphilis is known as 'The great imitator' in dermatology.
- Legal value-for migration to Gulf countries.
- As a work-up for connective tissue disorders specially lupus.

Semen Analysis

Ajinkya Gujrathi, Sanjeev Gupta, Rohit Singla

INTRODUCTION

- Semen is a fluid secreted from the accessory sex organs with suspension of spermatozoa, stored in the epididymis.
- About 90% of semen volume is made up of secretions from the accessory organs mainly the prostate and seminal vesicles, with minor contributions from the bulbourethral (Cowper's) glands and epididymis. Hormonal control of Spermatogenesis is depicted in **Flowchart 1**.
- Freshly-ejaculated semen is a coagulum that liquefies over a 5–25-minute time period. Semen is formed by:
  - Urethral glands (2–4%)
  - Prostate (20–30%): Secretion contain citrate, zinc, acid phosphatase and proteolytic enzymes
  - Seminal vesicles (46–80%): It is rich in fructose, vitamin C, prostaglandin and protein kinase
  - Testis and epididymis (5–10%): Alpha-glucosidase isoenzyme

Indications for semen analysis:
- As an investigation of infertility
- To know whether a vasectomy or vasectomy reversal has been successful (usually done 6 weeks after the vasectomy)
- To check patency of the male ducts and the function of the accessory glands
- To support or disprove a denial of paternity on the grounds of sterility
- In medicolegal cases
- For selection of sperm donors for artificial insemination

Semen collection: Testing is recommended after a period of abstinence of 2–7 days. Preferably two or three samples needed for conclusive report. Different methods used for semen collection are:
- Masturbation
- Condom collection
- Epididymal extraction

The sample should never be obtained through coitus interruptus for following reasons:
- Some part of ejaculation could be lost
- Bacterial contamination of sample could occur
- Low (acidic) vaginal pH could adversely affect sperm motility

Quality of semen specimen varies depending on how the ejaculate is produced, e.g., the ejaculate produced by masturbation and collected into containers in a room near the laboratory can be of lower quality than those recovered from nonspermicidal condoms used during intercourse at home. That's why in certain circumstances, collection of

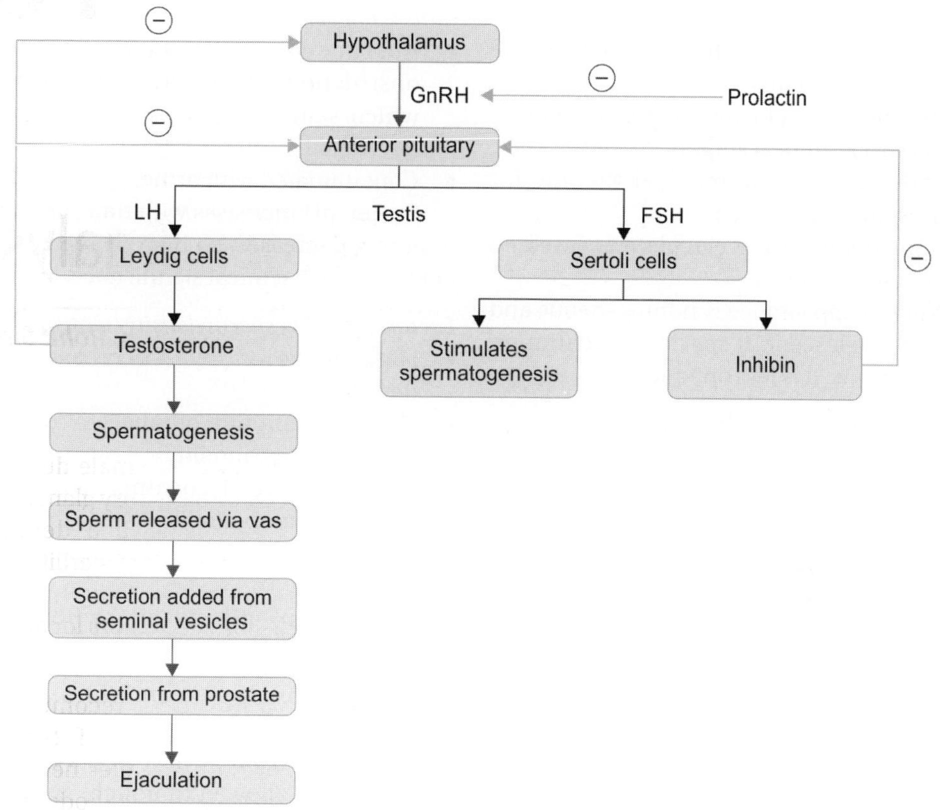

FLOWCHART 1: Hormonal control of spermatogenesis.
(GnRH: gonadotropin-releasing hormone; LH: luteinizing hormone; FSH: follicle-stimulating hormone)

semen at home can also be done provided the collected sample is delivered to the laboratory within 1 hour and during transport; sample should be kept between 20 and 37°C.

The semen sample should be ideally examined within 30 minutes to 1 hour of collection, to prevent dehydration or changes in temperature from affecting semen quality. The optimal sexual abstinence for semen sample obtaining is from 2 to 7 days.

A routine semen analysis should include:
- Physical characteristics of semen (color, odor, pH, viscosity and liquefaction)
- Volume
- Concentration
- Morphology
- Sperm motility

Postejaculate Urinalysis

The presence of sperm in the urine is called retrograde ejaculation.

There are two potential sources for sperm in the postejaculate urinalysis (PEU):
1. True retrograde ejaculation of sperm into the bladder
2. Incomplete emptying of semen from the urethra with washing out of residual sperm containing semen during subsequent urination

Indications of PEU:
- Diabetic patients with low semen volume and sperm counts
- Patients with a history of pelvic, bladder or retroperitoneal surgery
- Patients receiving medical therapy for prostatic enlargement
- Appearance of the ejaculate is assessed after liquefaction
- Normal appearance is homogeneous and gray-opalescent. If sperm concentration is very low, it is less opaque.

The color may also be different:
- Slightly yellow—prolonged abstinence
- Deep yellow—pyospermia, jaundice or taking certain vitamins or drugs
- Red-brown—red blood cells are present (hemospermia)
  - Trauma to the genital tract
  - Inflammation
  - Tumor of the genital tract
- Rust color—small bleedings in seminal vesicles

Volume: Semen volumes between 2 and 5 mL are normal; as per World Health Organization (WHO) 1.5 mL is taken as the lower reference limit. Ejaculate is mostly composed of water 96–98%. So, the poor water intake may cause reduction in ejaculate volume.

Causes of low semen volume are:
- Obstruction of the ejaculatory duct
- Congenital bilateral absence of the vas deferens (CBAVD)
- Partial retrograde ejaculation
- Androgen deficiency
- Inadequate erection and improper mood at collection
- Incomplete collection

High semen volume: It may reflect active exudation in cases of active inflammation of the accessory organs.

Normal pH value ≥ 7.2

Causes of pH < 7.0:
- Absence of sperm ejaculatory duct obstruction or CBAVD, a condition in which seminal vesicles are also poorly developed.
- Contaminated with urine.

Semen pH increases with time, as natural buffering decreases, so high pH values may not have much clinical significance.

Factors affecting sperm density/motility:
- High intake of soya—decrease sperm density
- High consumption of tobacco—decrease sperm density/motility
- Consumption of cocaine/marijuana—decrease sperm motility
- Vaginal lubricants—decrease sperm motility
- Alcoholism—affects all semen parameters

Semen microscopy examination: After collecting the sample as described above, the physical examination is carried out. The sample is allowed to liquefy as it is not possible to make smear on coagulated semen sample. There is an enzyme secreted by semen vesicle called protein kinase, which keeps it coagulated, during ejaculation some enzymes are secreted by prostate which cause liquefaction of the semen. So, prostatic problem may cause delayed liquefaction and uncoagulated sample may denote a seminal vesicle pathology.

After liquefaction, two smears are prepared, one direct smear for sperm morphology and another one for sperm count. At least five fields and 200 sperms are examined. The sperm motility can be graded from grade A-D. Highly motile sperms cross out from coverslip and go away. The morphological study of spermatozoa is possible only on high resolution. On detailed microscopic examination clumping of sperms can be seen which can be of head to head, tail to tail

TABLE 1: Normal parameters.

Parameters	Range	Abnormalities
Ejaculate volume	1.5–4.5 mL	• Aspermia—absence of semen • Hypospermia—semen volume < 1.5 mL • Hyperspermia—semen volume > 4.5 mL
Sperm concentration	15–259 m/mL	• Azoospermia—absence of sperm in semen • Oligospermia—low sperm count • Polyzoospermia—high sperm concentration > 200 m/mL
Total motility	40–81%	Asthenozoospermia—no motile sperm/decreased motility
Vitality (live spermatozoa)	58% or more	Necrozoospermia—dead sperms
Sperm morphology (% of normal forms)	4–48%	Teratozoospermia—abnormal morphology of sperms (shape), caused by either defect in the head, midpiece, and/or tail

Notes:
- Leukocyte counts/red blood cell (RBC)—almost nil. Not more than 1×10^6/mL.
- As per World Health Organization (WHO) 2010 guidelines, over 15 million sperm per mL is considered normal. But as per older definition this value was 20 million.

or mixed type. This clumping may indirectly denote antisperm antibodies.

The sperm count is done on Neubauer chamber. Normal parameters of semen analysis are listed in **Table 1**.

EXAMINATION IN CASE OF OLIGOSPERMIA/AZOOSPERMIA

Physical Examination

Testis:
- Size
- Position (cryptorchid)
- Volume (normal ~15–25 mL)
- Firmness (normal = firm)—a soft and/or small testis is indicative of abnormal spermatogenesis

Vas deferens: Bilateral congenital absence of vas deferens (CAVD) suggests Wolffian duct anomalies while unilateral absence may be associated with renal agenesis.

Epididymis: The epididymis is typically difficult to appreciate.

Investigations

Semen fructose testing is indicated in men with low ejaculate volumes and no sperm. It helps in assessing level of obstruction.

Normal value = 120–450 mg%

It is absent in:
- Seminal vesicle agenesis
- Ductal obstruction
- Congenital bilateral absence of the vas deferens

Antisperm antibodies (ASAs): Up to 5–10% of male infertility attributed to ASAs in men. These are seen in 10% of infertile and 3% of fertile men.

Etiology:
- Injury to blood-testis barrier
- Obstruction (postvasectomy reversal)
- Infection (orchitis)
- Trauma/torsion
- Varicocele/cryptorchidism

Testing indications: Decreased motility and sperm agglutination (on smear head to head, tail to tail clumping)

Available tests:

- *Direct*: It detects sperm-bound immuno-globulins
- *Indirect*: It detects biologic activity of circulating ASA
- Enzyme-linked immunosorbent assay (ELISA)
- Others (flow cytometry and radiolabeled)
- *Blood tests*: Blood glucose, thyroid function test (TFT), liver function test (LFT), prolactin, follicle stimulating hormone/luteinizing hormone (FSH/LH), testosterone, and prostate-specific antigen (PSA) in some cases. Correlation of testosterone, LH, FSH and prolactin with clinical presentation is given in **Table 2**.

Direct (on sperm) is more valid than indirect (serum, mucus and seminal plasma) ASA test.

Abdominal ultrasonography (USG): To assess for kidneys in cases with absent vas deferens.

- Ipsilateral renal anomalies—80% cases with unilateral absence of vas deferens

- Renal agenesis—most common
  - 25% unilateral absence of vas deferens
  - 10% CBAVD

Scrotal USG:

- To assess for varicocele only in patients with inadequate physical examination such as obese patients
- To detect testicular tumors in patients with suggestive history, examination or hormonal values

Vasography is the gold standard test for assessing the patency of the male ductal system. It is indicated for determination of the site of obstruction in the azoospermic patient with confirmed normal spermatogenesis on testis biopsy. It is currently rarely performed because image modalities such as transrectal ultrasound (TRUS) and magnetic resonance imaging (MRI) have superseded it.

Testicular biopsy/fine needle aspiration cytology (FNAC):

- Site—medial or lateral surface of the upper pole.
- In presence of marked elevation (≥ 2 times of normal) of FSH, testicular biopsy is indicated only if sperm retrieval with intracytoplasmic sperm injection (ICSI) is being considered.

Chips for home use are emerging that can give an accurate estimation of sperm count after three samples taken on different days.

Computer-assisted semen analysis (CASA): The computer calculates sperm motility, sperm concentration, total sperm count and the percentage of motile spermatozoa in the sample. CASA cannot accurately predict "fertility" that will be obtained with a semen sample or subject.

Semen samples may vary from day to day, 2 or 3 samples within a 3–6 months period may be evaluated for accurate testing.

TABLE 2: Correlation of testosterone, LH, FSH, and prolactin with clinical presentation.				
Presentation	**FSH**	**LH**	**Testosterone**	**Prolactin**
Normal spermatogenesis	N	N	N	N
Hypogonadotropic hypogonadism	↓	↓	↓	N
Abnormal spermatogenesis	↑/N	N	N	N
Complete testicular failure hypergonadotropic/hypogonadism	↑	↑	N/↓	N
Hyperprolactinemia-pituitary tumor	N/↓	N/↓	↓	↑

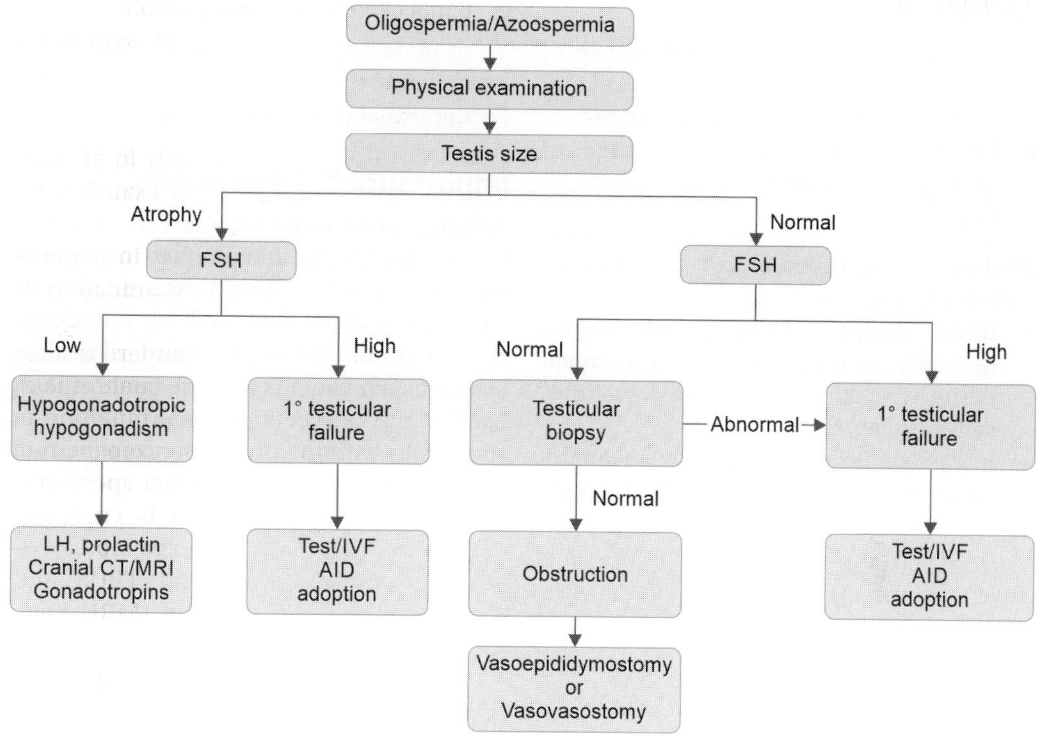

FLOWCHART 2: Approach to a case of oligospermia/azoospermia.
(AID: artificial insemination by donor; CT: computed tomography; FSH: follicle stimulating hormone; IVF: in vitro fertilization; LH: luteinizing hormone; MRI: magnetic resonance imaging; TESE: testicular sperm extraction)

Limitation of Semen Analysis

- It is impossible to characterize a man's semen quality from evaluation of a single semen sample. So it is helpful to examine two or three samples to obtain baseline data
- Normal semen analysis may not reflect the true fertility status of an individual
- Only 50% of subfertile men have recognizable causes detectable by semen analysis

Causes of Oligospermia/ Azoospermia

- *Pretesticular*:
  - Hypothalamic pituitary disorders:
    - Congenital causes—Kallmann syndrome and hemochromatosis
    - Acquired causes—tumors, trauma, postsurgery, systemic diseases and drugs like gonadotropin-releasing hormone (GnRH) agonists
- *Testicular causes*:
  - Congenital causes—Klinefelter syndrome, cryptorchidism, varicocele and anorchia
  - Acquired causes—trauma, torsion, castration, viral orchitis, systemic diseases like renal failure, hepatic cirrhosis, etc., ionizing radiation and drugs such as ketoconazole, spironolactone, antiandrogens, etc.
- *Post-testicular*:
  - Epididymal dysfunction because of drugs or infection

- - Vas deferens abnormalities
  - Ejaculatory dysfunction because of spinal cord disease, premature ejaculation and autonomic dysfunction
- Idiopathic (approach to a case of oligospermia/azoospermia is given in **Flowchart 2**)

Medicolegal significance of detection of semen/sperms.
- Rape, sodomy (anal intercourse), bestiality (sexual intercourse by a human being with a lower animal like dogs, calves, sheep, etc.)
- In case of false accusation by a woman, incest (sexual intercourse in blood relation) and sexual murders.

- Semen is the second most common form of material tested for DNA. It is almost certainly the primary evidence in most of the sexual crimes such as rape.

Importance in Dermatology

Semen analysis is not a primary investigation for a dermatologist, but many times patients with psycho-sexual disorders and infertility can present in the OPD. So basic knowledge of semen analysis is necessary to treat or counsel such patients as these patients keep oscillating between doctors of different specialties without any proper treatment or counselling.

Antibodies in Autoimmune Connective Tissue Disease

Sunita Gupta, Sanjeev Gupta

AUTOANTIBODIES IN CONNECTIVE TISSUE DISORDERS

Before discussing auto-antibodies, we must first understand what is immunity and auto-immunity.

Immunity and autoimmunity—the human body has many defence mechanisms against pathogens, one of which is humoral immunity. This defence mechanism produces antibodies (large glycoproteins) in response to an immune stimulus. Many cells of the immune system are required for this process, including lymphocytes (T-cells and B-cells) and antigen presenting cells (APCs). These cells coordinate an immune response upon detection of foreign proteins (antigen), producing antibodies that bind to these antigens. In normal physiology, lymphocytes that recognize human proteins (autoantigens) either undergo programmed cell death (apoptosis) or become non-functional.

This self-tolerance (**Fig. 1**) indicates that lymphocytes should not incite an immune response against human cellular antigens. At times loss of tolerance, due to defects at single/multiple levels of immune regulation, autoantibodies are produced against various components of cells. These antibodies act on their specific targets leading to stimulation of immune cascade, they are deposited on respective cellular components and cause destruction of tissue. Meaning thereby, our own body cells are being attacked by immune cells. This process is called autoimmunity and is responsible for autoimmune diseases. The antibodies can be formed against any cellular components.

Self-tolerance

There are two types of tolerance: (i) central tolerance and (ii) peripheral tolerance.

Central tolerance: Works at the level of primary lymphoid organs (bone marrow, thymus) via following mechanisms:
- Negative selection
- Generation of regulatory T-cells

Peripheral tolerance: Works at the level of peripheral tissues via following mechanisms:
- Clonal anergy
- Clonal deletion
- Regulatory T-cells
- T-T interaction

The major antibodies are as follows:
- Antibodies to phospholipid (cardiolipin) [antiphospholipid antibodies (APLA)]—against phospholipid component of cell wall
- Antineutrophilic cytoplasmic antibodies (ANCA)—against cytoplasmic components of neutrophils
- Antimitochondrial antibodies—against mitochondria

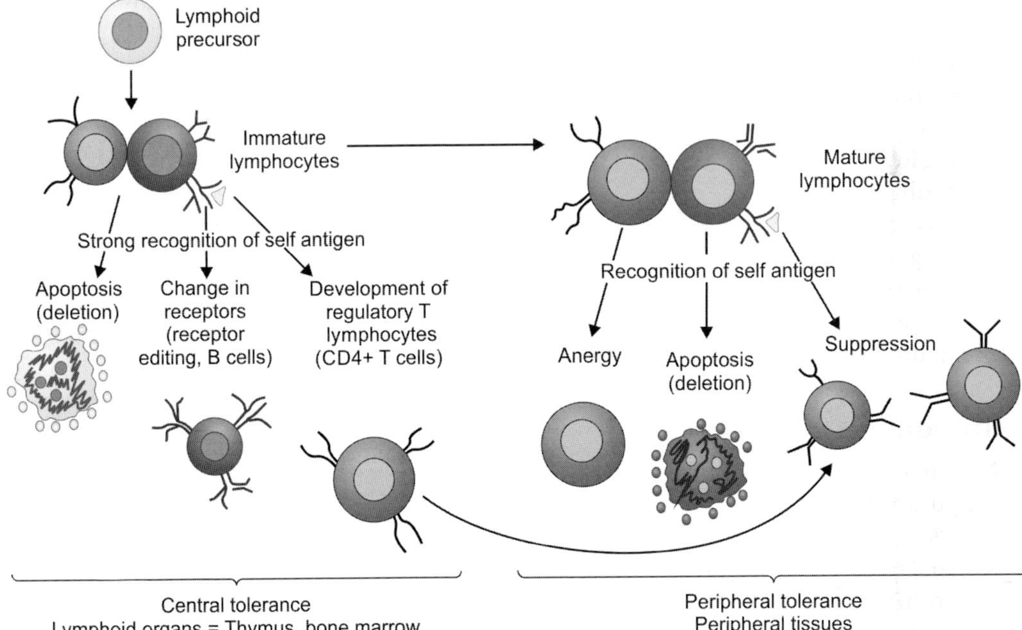

FIG. 1: Mechanisms of central and peripheral tolerance.

- Antinuclear antibodies (ANA)*—against nucleus:
  - Antibodies against deoxyribonucleic acid (DNA):
    - Antibodies to double stranded DNA (dsDNA)
    - Antibodies to single stranded (ssDNA)
  - Antibodies against nonhistone proteins bound to ribonucleic acid (RNA):
    - Antibodies to Ro (SS-A)
    - Antibodies to La (SS-B)
    - Antibodies to U1RNP
    - Antibodies to Sm
- Antibodies to histones
- Antibodies to centromere
- Antichromatin
- Anti-RNA polymerase III (known as ARA)
- Serum antitopoisomerase (also known as Scl-70)
- Anti Jo-1

ANTIPHOSPHOLIPID ANTIBODIES

- *Association*: SLE (50%) and SCLE (10–16%)
- *APLAs mainly consist of 3 subtypes of antibodies*: Lupus anticoagulant, anticardiolipin antibody, beta-2 glycoprotein 1. Most of the laboratories perform testing of all these three antibodies in combination, whenever APLA testing is advised, however, the individual testing and titer is also available, but costly.

---

*The term ANA is a broad term, they can be directed against any component of nucleus or enzyme, e.g., double stranded DNA, single stranded DNA, RNA, histone protein, nucleolus, centromere, etc.

APLA IgM-up to 12U/mL-negative, 12-18U/mL-equivocal, more than 18U/mL-positive:

- Triple positivity indicate increased risk of development of APL syndrome.
- APLAs show cross reactivity in VDRL testing leading to false positive result.
- Cardiolipin antibody-associated with venous or arterial thrombosis
- Beta-2 glycoprotein 1 antibody-associated with recurrent fetal loss.
- Lupus anticoagulant-associated with premature births.

Indications for APLA Testing

- Livedo reticularis
- Purpura and necrosis
- Ulcers
- Internal organ thrombosis
- Recurrent miscarriages
- Screening in patients with SLE

ANTINEUTROPHIL CYTOPLASMIC ANTIBODY

Antineutrophil cytoplasmic antibody (ANCA) represent autoantibodies to inflammatory disorders. There are mainly 2 types of ANCA, i.e., cANCA and pANCA (some atypical forms are also there). There are mainly 2 enzymes in ANCA which take part in killing of bacteria:

- cANCA–or PR3-ANCA are a type of antibody against the antigen targets present in the cytoplasm of neutrophils. The most common target is proteinase 3 (PR3), hence the name.
- pANCA–or MPO-ANCA are a type of antibody that target the material around the nucleus of a neutrophil or perinuclear area. Most common target is myeloperoxidase (MPO), hence the name.

Formation of ANCA: The exact mechanism of formation of these antibodies is poorly understood. There are two theories proposed regarding this, namely theory of molecular mimicry and theory of defective apoptosis.

Indications for testing: In the evaluation of various vasculitic disorders like SLE, RA, primary biliary cirrhosis, Wegener's granulomatosis, Churg-Strauss, autoimmune hepatitis, MPA (microscopic polyangiitis).

ANCA can also be drug induced, e.g., Propylthiouracil, Ciprofloxacin, Sulfasalazine, Hydralazine, Pantoprazole, Minocycline, Allopurinol, D-penicillamine.

Antimitochondrial antibodies (AMAs) are immunoglobulins formed against mitochondria, primarily the mitochondria of liver cells. They are the characteristic markers of primary biliary cirrhosis (PBC). PBC causes scarring of liver tissue, confined primarily to the bile duct drainage system. AMA is present in about 95% of such cases. They are also associated with various types of myopathies but are not of much significance in dermatology.

Antichromatin antibodies are the major antibodies that lead to lupus erythematosus (LE) cell[#] formation. They are also known as LE cell factor, antinucleosome, anti-deoxyribonucleoprotein (DNP), etc. These autoantibodies are found in systemic lupus erythematosus (SLE) (75%), drug-induced lupus (100%) and autoimmune hepatitis (20–50%). Eukaryotic chromatin is comprised of approximately 40% DNA, 40% histones,

---

[#]Lupus erythematosus (LE) cell is a neutrophil or macrophage that has phagocytized (engulfed) the denatured nuclear material of another cell. LE cells should not be confused with Tart cells which have engulfed unaltered nuclei, but with a visible chromatin rather than homogeneous appearance.

20% nonhistone proteins [i.e., high mobility group (HMG) proteins], RNA, and other macromolecules. Therefore, antichromatin antibodies are somewhat similar to ANA. Perhaps the anti-chromatin is the older version of ANA.

ARA-Anti-RNA polymerase can be positive among anticentromere and anti-topoisomerase I (topo I) negative sera and serve as a marker of systemic sclerosis.

Anti-Jo: Although anti-Jo-1 antibodies are often included with ANAs, but they are actually antibodies to the cytoplasmic protein, *Histidyl-tRNA synthetase*—an aminoacyl-tRNA synthetase essential for the synthesis of histidine-loaded transfer ribonucleic acid (tRNA). They are highly associated with polymyositis and dermatomyositis, and are rarely found in other connective tissue diseases (CTD).

Antinuclear antibody is detected by indirect immunofluorescence test that utilizes a substrate rich in nuclear material or more recently used Hep-2 obtained from esophageal squamous cell carcinoma cells, available commercially, prefixed on glass slides.

American College of Rheumatology (ACR) recommendation:

"Do not test ANA subserologies without a positive ANA and clinical suspicion of immune-mediated disease".

- Ordering ANA subserologies before it is known that the ANA is positive—while potentially efficient for the clinician, such additional testing can be costly because tests for ANA subserologies (including antibodies to dsDNA, Sm, RNP, SSA, SSB, Scl-70, and centromere) are usually negative if the ANA is negative.
- There are important exceptions where subserology testing may be useful in the context of a negative ANA test. These include anti–Jo-1, which can be positive in a unique clinical subset of myositis, or sometimes, anti-SSA in the setting of lupus

or Sjögren's syndrome. Despite these exceptions, in most clinical situations, a stepwise approach (**Flowchart 1**) in which ANA subserologies are ordered only after an ANA is known to be positive is most appropriate.

Interpretation of results: ANA positivity is just a broad term; it is a screening test, not diagnostic for a specific disease. If ANA is positive, we have to know titer of the positive test, and the pattern of fluorescence and may need further tests [extractable nuclear antigens (ENA)] which are somewhat disease specific.

Methods of detection of ANA:
- Indirect immunofluorescence (IIF)-gold standard
- Enzyme-linked immunosorbent assay (ELISA)
- Immunodiffusion
- Counter immune electrophoresis (CIEP)
- Multiple immunobead assay

Sensitivity refers to the probability that a patient suggestive of having a CTD will have a positive serologic test result.

Specific serologic test is more likely to identify patients with a particular disease and exclude those without the disease. A test with a high specificity rules in, but does not rule out, a disease (**Table 1**).

ANA is a *sensitive test* as it can be positive in >95% of patients with SLE and is also detected in conjunction with CTDs. However, the ANA test *lacks specificity* and the presence of the antibody is not necessarily diagnostic for SLE.

Salient points regarding ANA testing:
- Titer-dilution after which the antibodies become undetectable
- Antinuclear antibody positivity by immunofluorescence test is useful only with titer
- A titer of 1:80 or less is of no diagnostic value (**Table 2**)

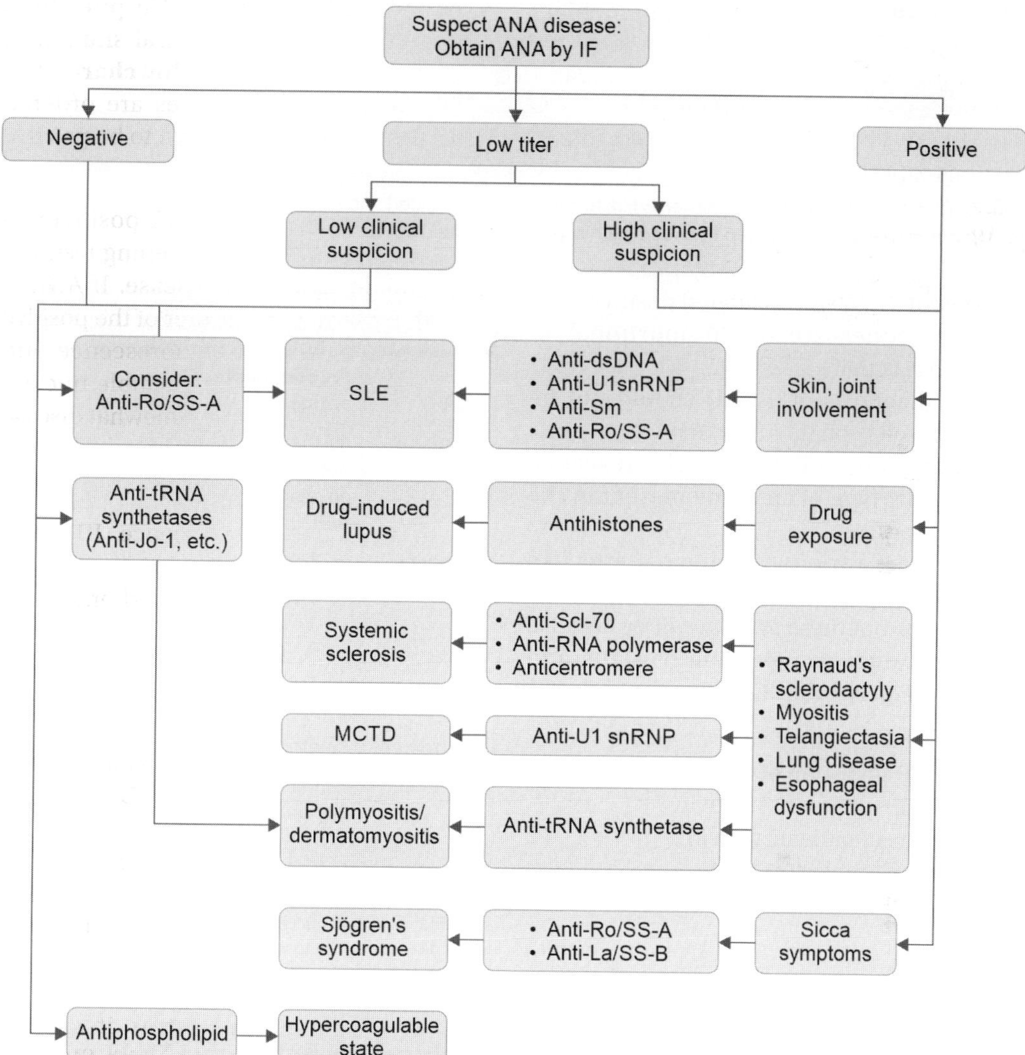

FLOWCHART 1: Approach and Interpretation of different auto-antibodies in a suspected case of connective tissue disorder.

TABLE 1: Sensitivity and specificity of ANA according to the method.

Method	ANA sensitivity	ANA specificity
IIF	80%	90–97%
ELISA	99%	36–94%

(ANA: antinuclear antibody; ELISA: enzyme-linked immuno-sorbent assay)

TABLE 2: Antinuclear antibody (ANA) titers and their prevalence in healthy general population.

Titer	Prevalence
1:40	32%
1:80	13%
1:160	5%
1:320	3%

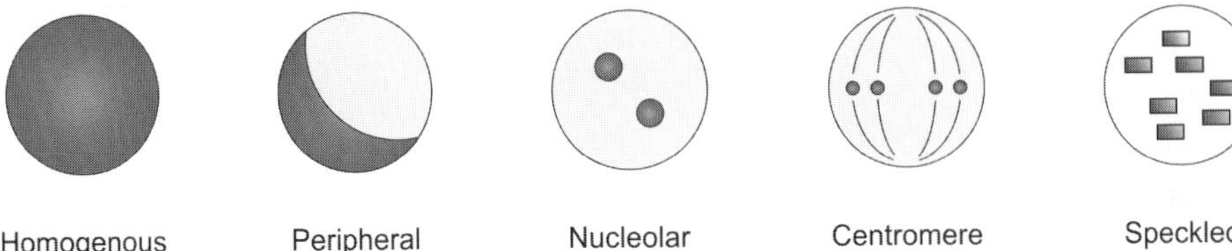

FIG. 2: There are various staining patterns like homogenous, speckled and localized to the centromere but these *lack specificity* because of overlap between staining patterns and diseases.

- Titer of ≥1:160 is considered positive
- Titer values are not proportional to disease activity
- The diagnosis of a CTD should not be made solely on titer of an ANA.

The pattern of nuclear fluorescence suggests the type of antibody present in the patient's serum.

There are various staining patterns like homogenous, speckled and localized to the centromere but these *lack specificity* because of overlap between staining patterns and diseases (**Fig. 2, Table 3**).

Indications for fluorescent ANA testing:
- Clinical suspicion of CTD
- Work-up for photosensitivity
- Baseline in patients with LE
- Baseline for phototherapy
- Work-up of chronic vasculitis

Conditions with positive ANA other than autoimmune diseases (false positive ANA):
- Elderly persons*
- Pregnant women
- Relatives of patients with CTD
- Other autoimmune diseases (e.g., PBC and autoimmune thyroiditis)
- Drugs (e.g., procainamide and hydralazine)
- Chronic infections
- Neoplasms
- Healthy persons

TABLE 3: Antinuclear antibody (ANA) patterns and their antigen and disease associations.		
ANA	**Predominant antigen**	**Disease**
Peripheral	dsDNA and nuclear envelope proteins	SLE
Homoge-neous	dsDNA and histones	SLE, RA, MCTD, and drug-induced lupus
Nucleolar	Nucleolar RNA	SSc, SLE, Sjögren's syndrome, and RA
Centromere	Kinetochore	CREST
Speckled	Various ribonu-cleoprotein	MCTD, SLE, SSc, and Sjögren's syndrome

(CREST: calcinosis, Raynaud's phenomenon, esophageal dysmotility, sclerodactyly, and telangiectasia; dsDNA: double stranded deoxyribonucleic acid; MCTD: mixed connective tissue disease; RA: rheumatoid arthritis; RNA: ribonucleic acid; SLE: systemic lupus erythematosus)

Antinuclear Antibody (ANA) Positivity in Various Connective Tissue Diseases

- Systemic lupus erythematosus (lupus or SLE)—over 95%
- Progressive systemic sclerosis (scleroderma)—60–90%
- Rheumatoid arthritis—25–30%

---

*Due to weakened immune function of clearance and elimination of self-reactive cells, ANA can be positive even in a healthy individuals. There can also be a genetic predisposition, infections, and tissue injury.

- Sjögren's syndrome (SS)—40–70%
- Mixed connective tissue disease (MCTD)—95%
- Juvenile arthritis—15–30%
- Drug-induced lupus—100%
- *Other causes*: Autoimmune hepatitis, polymyositis, dermatomyositis, Addison disease, idiopathic thrombocytopenic purpura, Hashimoto's thyroiditis, auto-immune hemolytic anemia, and type 1 diabetes mellitus.

ANTINUCLEAR ANTIBODY NEGATIVE SYSTEMIC LUPUS ERYTHEMATOSUS

- In case ANA testing is done on animal substrate.
- If the patient's ANA are solely against ssDNA. Because the fluorescent ANA substrate has intact nuclei without single strands of DNA, the test is expectedly negative.
- In some patients with photosensitivity and later reported as having subacute cutaneous lupus erythematosus (SCLE) with anti-Ro (SS-A) antibodies. They can have anticytoplasmic antibody, anti Ro/LA or anti-ssDNA antibody.

Antinuclear antibody sensitivity and speci-ficity in LE:
- For SLE, sensitivity is very high (98%)
- For SCLE 60–80%
- For discoid lupus erythematosus (DLE) 30–40%

ANTIBODIES TO DEOXYRIBONUCLEIC ACID

- In a eukaryotic cell, DNA is located in two locations, nucleus and mitochondria known as nDNA and mDNA respectively. Serum DNA antibody may recognize either double stranded DNA or single stranded DNA (dsDNA or ssDNA).
- The diagnostic significance of each of the two antibodies is different.
- Anti-nDNA testing technique using ELISA, radioimmunoassay, and IIF.
- Concentrated mitochondrial DNA (mDNA) is found within mitochondria and is called kinetoplast which is a double stranded, circular molecule containing 37 genes.
- Disease association-SLE (60%) and SCLE (10%).
- Other associations RA, Graves' disease, MCTD, SSc, and Sjögren disease.
- *Significance of anti-nDNA*:
  ○ Most frequently detected autoantibody associated with SLE.
  ○ Positive in 95% of patients of SLE with renal involvement.
  ○ Levels indicate lupus disease activity.
- Negative test does not rule out SLE.
- Single stranded DNA detected by ELISA, extracted nDNA are further denatured to produce ssDNA.
- Low diagnostic value for any CTD.
- Interpretation of result >3 standard deviations above the mean.

Extractable nuclear antigens: Extractable nuclear antigens are a group of autoantigens that were originally identified as antibody targets in people with autoimmune disorders. They are termed as ENA because they can be extracted from the cell nucleus with saline. ENAs consist of ribonucleoproteins (RNP) and nonhistone proteins, named by either the name of the donor who provided the prototype serum (Sm, Ro, La, and Jo), or the name of the disease setting in which the antibodies were found (SS-A, SS-B, and Scl-70).

The high specificity of these tests means that they should *only* be ordered in *ANA positive* patients with clinical features suggestive of a particular CTD and in ANA negative patients with known or suspected CTD.

These tests are intended for diagnostic confirmation but do not exclude a specific CTD.

These antibodies in general do not correlate with disease activity and, therefore, may be found in patients without active disease.

RIBONUCLEOPROTEIN ANTIBODY

- RNP or ribonucleoprotein is 1 of 4 auto-antigens commonly referred to as extractable nuclear antigens (ENA).
- Antibodies to RNP occur in approximately 50% of patients with lupus erythematosus (LE) and in patients with MCTD.
- Antibodies to various small nuclear ribonucleoprotein (snRNP) molecules are Ro (SS-A), La (SS-B), U1RNP, and Sm.
- *Detection technique:*
    - ○ Radioimmuno diffusion: High specificity and low sensitivity
    - ○ ELISA: High sensitivity and less specificity

Indications for anti-Ro (SS-A) and anti-La (SS-B) antibody testing: Anti-Ro and anti-La antibodies are named after the patient in which these were first discovered.
- Work-up for photosensitivity
- Screening for certain patients with LE
- Suspicion of subacute cutaneous LE
- Suspicion of neonatal LE
- Suspicion of Sjögren's syndrome
- Work-up for idiopathic chronic vasculitis
- Patients with systemic or subacute cutaneous LE with negative screening fluorescent ANA test.

Remarks
- Anti-Ro-strong association with photosensitivity (especially in SCLE), increased

TABLE 4: Incidence of anti-Ro (SS-A) antibodies in autoimmune connective tissue diseases (CTDs) by radial immunodiffusion.

Diagnosis	Percentage (%)
Antinuclear antibody negative SLE	70
Subacute cutaneous LE	70
Homozygous C2 or C4 deficiency	70
Late-onset SLE	80
Neonatal LE	95
Mothers of infants with neonatal LE	95
Discoid LE	0–20
Sjögren's syndrome	50
SSc and dermatomyositis	Rare
Healthy persons	<1

(LE: lupus erythematosus; SLE: systemic lupus erythematosus)

risk of congenital heart block, high incidence of vasculitis, and lower risk of nephritis (**Table 4**).
- Anti-La-associated with late onset SLE, secondary Sjögren's syndrome, neonatal lupus syndrome, anti-Ro antibodies and a lower risk for nephritis.

ANTIBODIES TO U1 RIBONUCLEOPROTEIN (U1-RNP) AND ANTISMITH (ANTI-Sm)

- *U1RNP:* Antinuclear RNP (anti-nRNP) antibodies, also known as anti-U1-RNP antibodies are very characteristic of MCTD (100%), can be positive in SLE (30%), and SCLE (10%).
- Presence of anti-U1RNP antibody is usually associated with sclerodactyly, Raynaud phenomenon, esophageal dysmotility, low incidence of renal disease, pulmonary dysfunction, arthritis, and myositis. Anti-U1RNP are often found with anti-Smith (anti-Sm) antibodies.

- Anti-Smith antibodies are a very specific marker for SLE. They are associated with central nervous system involvement, kidney disease, lung fibrosis, and pericarditis in SLE. It is not associated with disease activity. Highly diagnostic of SLE, however, sensitivity is low (15–40%). The antigens of the anti-Sm antibodies are the core units of the small nuclear RNPs (snRNPs).

Ant-dsDNA and anti-Sm are specific to SLE but only anti-dsDNA correlates with disease activity and with occurrence of glomerulonephritis. The dsDNA is more sensitive therefore more preferred.

ANTIHISTONE ANTIBODIES

- Histone is basic proteins that bind DNA strand and contribute to the supercoil formation.
- Characteristic of drug-induced SLE (90%), idiopathic SLE (30%) and resolves after several weeks of discontinuation of medications.
- *Drugs causing LE like disease*:
  - Antiarrhythmic: Procainamide, disopyramide, and propafenone
  - Antitubercular: Isoniazid and rifampicin
  - Antiepileptic: Carbamazepine and phenytoin
  - Neuroleptics such as chlorpromazine and lithium
  - Antithyroid drug: Propylthiouracil
  - Antihypertensives: Captopril, acebutolol/atenolol, diltiazem, and hydralazine
  - Others: Sulfasalazine, lovastatin, simvastatin, interferon (IFN), tumor necrosis factor (TNF) (I), minocycline, tetracycline, penicillamine, tiotropium bromide inhaler, ophthalmic timolol, etc.

ANTICENTROMERE

Anticentromere antibodies are autoantibodies specific to centromere part of chromosome. They occur in limited systemic scleroderma (60%) [formerly called CREST (calcinosis, Raynaud's phenomenon, esophageal dysmotility, sclerodactyly, and telangiectasia) syndrome], and occasionally in the diffuse form of scleroderma (15%). They are rare in other rheumatic conditions and in healthy people.

The specificity of this test is >98%. Thus, a positive anticentromere antibody finding is strongly suggestive of limited systemic scleroderma. Anticentromere antibodies present early in the course of disease and are notably predictive of limited cutaneous involvement and a decreased likelihood of aggressive internal organ involvement such as fibrosis in the lungs.

ANTITOPOISOMERASE (ANTI-Scl-70)

Anti-Scl-70 (also called antitopoisomerase I after the type I topoisomerase target) is an antitopoisomerase antibody-type of ANA, seen mainly in diffuse systemic scleroderma (with a sensitivity of 28–70%), but is also seen in 10–18% cases of limited form of systemic scleroderma. Anti-Scl-70 antibodies are associated with more severe scleroderma disease.

The etymology of Scl-70 consists of an abbreviation of scleroderma and a 70 kD extractable immunoreactive fragment that can be obtained from the otherwise larger (100–105 kD) target topoisomerase antigen (called the Scl-70 antigen) of the antibodies (**Table 5**).

DERMATOMYOSITIS

Myositis-associated antibodies (MAAs) are antibodies that occur in myositis but are not

TABLE 5: Different antibodies in scleroderma.

Reactivity	Target antigen	Frequency
Centromere	CENP proteins	60% LcSSc 2% DcSSc
SCL 70	Topoisomerase	40% Dc 15% Lc
RNAP	RNA polymerase 111	25% Dc 2% Lc
NRNP	U1RNP	15% SSc
PM-SCL		15% SSc

TABLE 6: Different antibodies associated with myositis.

Antibody	Prevalence	Significance
155 kD/Se	20–80%	Classic DM and amyopathic
140 kD	53%	Clinical amyopathic DM
Jo1	20%	PM, fever, ILD, RP, MH, and antisynthetase syndrome
Mi-2	15%	Shawl sign, prominent, and cuticular changes
ANA (speckled and nucleolar)	40%	Clinical amyopathic DM

(DM: dermatomyositis; ILD: interstitial lung disease; PM: polymyositis; RP: Raynaud's phenomenon)

specific for it. Anti-52kD Ro antibodies are the most common MAA. Some other examples are anti-Ku, anti-U1-RNP, U3-RNP and PM-Scl antibodies.

Myositis-specific antibodies (MSA) are specific for myositis and help define phenotype (**Table 6**). MSAs are:
- *Anti-Jo-1*: This is the most common type.
- Anti-MDA-5 antibodies are associated with a distinctive cutaneous phenotype characterized by vasculopathic ulcers on the fingers, knuckles, elbows and knees and painful red papules on the palmar surfaces of the metacarpophalangeal and interphalangeal joints. These are associated with a high incidence of clinically amyopathic disease (CADM) and interstitial lung disease (ILD).
- Anti-TIF-1γ antibodies are specific to dermatomyositis (DM) and are found in around 15–20% of cases. They are associated with severe skin disease and a high incidence of cancer. So these patients need a thorough screen for malignancy.
- Anti-NXP2 antibodies are frequent in Juvenile DM where they are associated with calcinosis while these are rare in adults.
- Anti-Mi-2 antibodies are specific to DM and are found in around 10–20% of cases. Patients with this antibody generally have classic cutaneous features of DM while muscle disease tends to be mild and ILD is rare in patients with these antibodies.
- Anti-SUMO-activating enzyme antibodies occur in 8% of adult DM patients.

Take Home Message/Importance in Dermatology

- Connective tissue disorders are misdiagnosed or over-diagnosed by general physicians very often.
- Skin being the accessory and the largest organ, the antibodies involve the skin in most of connective tissue disorders, so the role of Dermatologist is very important in early diagnosis and proper interpretation of various immunological tests.
- ANA is an important screening test, though it lacks specificity (**Flowchart 1**).
- There are specific antibodies for a specific connective tissue disorders but most of the time there is an overlap or coexistence of other antibodies without the proper, classical features of that particular

TABLE 7: Different antibodies in common connective tissue disorders.

Disease	nDNA	Sm	U1RNP	Ro (SS-A)	La (SS-B)	Centromere	Scl-70	Histone
SLE	+	+	–	–	–	–	–	–
MCTD	–	–	+	–	–	–	–	–
SS and SCLE	–	–	–	+	+	–	–	–
Ssc and CREST	–	–	–	–	–	+	+	–
Drug LE	–	–	–	–	–	–	–	+

(CREST: calcinosis, Raynaud's phenomenon, esophageal dysmotility, sclerodactyly, and telangiectasia; DNA: deoxyribonucleic acid; LE: lupus erythematosus; MCTD: mixed connective tissue disease; SCLE: subacute cutaneous lupus erythematosus; SLE: systemic lupus erythematosus; SS: Sjögren's syndrome)

disorder. Such patients may not have any clinical significance of antibodies detected, but they should be kept under observation for development of any new clinical features or change in titer of antibodies present (**Table 7**).

- Every antibody has its specific interpretation which may indicate disease activity or involvement of a particular organ and can predict disease outcome or prognosis.

C-reactive Protein

Rohit Batra, Nidhi Jindal

INTRODUCTION

C-reactive protein (CRP) is a protein found in blood plasma. The level rises in response to any kind of inflammation. The name CRP was given as it was first identified as a substance in the serum of patients with acute inflammation that reacted with the "c" carbohydrate antibody of the capsule of pneumococcus.

It is an acute-phase protein also called acute phase reactant, synthesized by liver, it rises following interleukin-6 secretion by macrophages and T cells. It binds to lysophosphatidylcholine expressed on the surface of dead or dying cells (and some types of bacteria) in order to activate the complement system. It rises more in bacterial infections as compared to viral infections. So, sometimes it may help in differentiating viral and bacterial infections, but many patients of COVID-19 also had increased CRP which may be due to superadded bacterial infection rather than viral inflammation.

Acute-phase protein (APP) or acute phase reactants: These are the class of proteins whose plasma concentration increases (positive APP) or decrease (negative APP) in response to inflammation. APP are produced by hepatocytes, and may be extrahepatic synthesis by epithelial cells, endothelial cells, and connective tissue, e.g., fibroblast adipocytes. Levels change approximately 1–2 hours for 1–2 days after onset of a systemic inflammatory reaction or other stimuli.

Positive APPs: CRP, serum amyloid A (SAA), ceruloplasmin, ferritin, α2 macroglobulin, fibrinogen, and complement (C3/C4).

Negative APPs: Albumin, transferrin, transthyretin, and retinol binding protein (RBP).

Functions of CRP:
- *Anti-infective*:
  - Opsonize particles for phagocytosis
  - Activate complement via classical pathway
- *Anti-inflammatory actions*:
  - C-reactive protein aids in the release of neutrophils from blood vessels, while preventing white cell adhesion to vessel in noninflamed tissue
  - Stimulate release of anti-inflammatory molecules from monocytes

FACTOR AFFECTING C-REACTIVE PROTEIN LEVELS

- *Gender*: Women have higher levels than men
- *Body mass effect*: Weight loss causes decrease in CRP

- *Ethnicity*: Blacks have higher levels than whites
- *Exercise*: After exercise CRP levels decrease
- *Alcohol consumption*: Decreases CRP

Methods for detection of CRP:
- Enzyme-linked immunosorbent assay (ELISA)
- Immunoturbidimetry
- Rapid immunodiffusion
- Visual agglutination

CLINICAL IMPORTANCE OF C-REACTIVE PROTEIN

- C-reactive protein levels are marker of acute and chronic inflammation and may help in determining response to treatment or disease severity. Since CRP is mainly produced by liver cells, so, liver damage may decrease CRP levels. In case of viral infections, there is production of interferon-alpha which is an inhibitor of CRP production leading to relatively low levels of CRP as compared to bacterial infections.
- As compared to the erythrocyte sedimentation rate, which is an indirect test for inflammation, the levels of CRP rise and fall rapidly with the onset and removal of the inflammatory stimulus, respectively. More modest elevations tend to be associated with a broader spectrum of etiologies, ranging from sleep disturbances to periodontal disease.

Elevated CRP levels:
- Osteoarthritis
- Predictive of coronary events (especially in stable angina)
- Proinflammatory or prothrombotic effects
- *Mild elevation of CRP levels*: Systemic lupus erythematosus (SLE), scleroderma, Sjogren syndrome, and dermatomyositis/polymyositis

- *Normalization of CRP levels*: Helpful tool in determining the response to antibiotic therapy and duration of treatment
- *Transplant cases*: Elevated levels were seen in majority of kidney or heart transplant—highly elevated in graft-versus-host disease (GVHD)—changes in levels are not organ specific like other inflammatory conditions
- *Cerebral vein or sinus thrombosis*: An increase CRP is associated with a poorer short-term prognosis
- Giant cell arteritis
- Pancreatitis

Interpretations of blood levels:
- *<0.3 mg/dL*: Normal level seen in healthy adults
- *0.3–1.0 mg/dL*: Normal or minor elevation—obesity, sedentary lifestyle, depression, pregnancy, diabetes, common cold, periodontitis, gingivitis, and cigarette smoking
- *1–10.0 mg/dL*: Moderate elevation—rheumatoid arthritis (RA), SLE or other autoimmune diseases, myocardial infarction, bronchitis, malignancies, and pancreatitis
- *More than 10.0 mg/dL*: Marked elevation—acute bacterial infections, systemic vasculitis, major trauma, and sometimes in acute viral infections
- *More than 50.0 mg/dL*: Severe elevation—acute bacterial infections

Importance in dermatology:
- As a marker of underlying infection specially when patient needs steroids and immunosuppressant.
- As a marker for severity of inflammation in work up, treatment, follow-up cases of psoriatic arthritis, Reiters, CTD, etc.
- Another dermatologic disease associated with elevations in CRP is chronic spontaneous urticaria. Multiple studies demonstrated that circulating levels of

IL-6 and CRP are significantly elevated in patients with chronic urticaria, and the increase in levels corresponded to the severity and activity of the disease.

- Elevated levels of CRP are a marker of cancer risk in healthy individuals. A recent study reported an association of nonmelanoma skin cancer with elevated plasma CRP.
- Elevated plasma CRP levels were also observed in association with inflammatory acne lesions.
- CRP is a nonspecific test and was not commonly prescribed till COVID era. In COVID, CRP was very frequently prescribed. The high levels of CRP seen in cases of COVID were because of superadded bacterial infection or viral infection per se, will remain a mystery and will be difficult to solve in future.

Rheumatoid Factor

Rohit Batra, Sanjeev Gupta

INTRODUCTION

- Rheumatoid factor (RF) has been known to be one of the characteristics of rheumatoid arthritis (RA) and has been used to diagnose, classify, and characterize patients with this disease. It is still the most widely used serological marker of RA, and one of the seven criteria of the American College of Rheumatology for classification of RA.
- Rheumatoid factors are immunoglobulins (Ig) that bind the Fc (constant region) of IgG. This part of the molecule is essential for complement fixation and interaction with the Fc receptor, and thus for uptake of immune complexes. RFs of all subtypes can be seen in the earliest stages of the disease and can precede the onset of RA by several years. The major RF species is the IgM isotype, while IgG- and IgA-RF occur less frequently.
- Immunoglobulin M-RF can be detected in 60–80% of RA patients with established disease, while prevalence in patients with early RA is usually <50%. IgM-RF is an important tool that helps the clinician in making a diagnosis as well as in decisions regarding therapeutic measures.
- Interestingly, IgA-RF appears to be a more specific marker antibody for RA than IgM- or IgG-RF. The clinical specificity of IgA RF is not clear, but it has been found early in the course of rheumatoid arthritis. IgA RF, probably from the mucosae, is the most common isotype in Sjogren's syndrome.
- But RF is not pathognomonic for RA and frequently occurs in other disorders as well as in healthy individuals.
- Commonly used cut-off value is 15 or 20 IU/mL, IgM-RF shows only moderate specificity for RA. High-titer RF (RF 50 IU/mL), in contrast, has been shown to be highly discriminative between RA and non-RA in patients with early arthritis.

The sensitivity of RF for established rheumatoid arthritis is only 60–70% with a specificity of 78%.

Probably even more importantly, RF also gives some prognostic information as it is associated with:

- Erosive disease
- More rapid progression of joint destruction
- Persistence of arthritis
- Extra-articular manifestations
- Worse outcome.

The association of high-titer RF with more severe disease further point toward pathogenetic role of RFs.

The detection of RF has been a key diagnostic tool in the diagnosis of RA.

Conventional assays detect IgM RF, but IgG and IgA RF can be detected using specialized assays.

METHODS OF DETECTION

- Rose–Waller test, which relies on the ability of RFs to agglutinate sheep erythrocytes coated with anti-sheep Ig.
- Latex agglutination test—in which latex particles coated with human IgG aggregate in the presence of IgM RF (>20 IU/mL). These tests identify only the IgM isotype.
- Detection of IgG and IgA RF by enzyme-linked immunosorbent assay (ELISA) is not widely used in practice as it is expensive.
- Quantitative tests are also available for RF, it is done in serial dilutions of the serum (1:10, 1:20, 1:30 and so on), which indicate RF concentration 40, 80, 120 IU/mL respectively.

Diseases in which elevated RF is seen:
- Rheumatoid arthritis
- Systemic lupus erythematosus (SLE)
- Sjögren's syndrome (60%)
- Chronic osteomyelitis
- 10% of the general population especially the elderly
- Hepatitis B
- Hepatitis C virus (HCV)-associated cryoglobulinemia
- Tuberculosis
- Syphilis
- Leishmaniasis

Rheumatoid factor is more sensitive for RA but not specific. Anti-CCP is more specific.

If patient has symptoms of rheumatoid arthritis, and the results show:
- Positive CCP antibodies and positive RF, it likely means that the patient has rheumatoid arthritis.
- Positive CCP antibodies and negative RF, it may mean that patient is in the early stages of rheumatoid arthritis or will develop it in the future.
- Negative CCP antibodies and negative RF, it means that patient is less likely to have rheumatoid arthritis.

Importance in dermatology:
- To evaluate a case of Psoriatic arthritis. RA should be negative in psoriasis.
- As a work-up for CTD.

Anti-cyclic Citrullinated Peptide

Rohit Batra, Sanjeev Gupta

INTRODUCTION

Dying or degenerating cells produce an enzyme known as peptidyl arginine-deaminase (PAD). This enzyme acts on certain arginine containing extracellular proteins leading to formation of a nonstandard amino acid known as citrulline. This whole process is known as citrullination which is a normal physiological process associated with cell death.

Normally, citrulline containing proteins are present in brain and keratin layer of epidermis. In some pathological states of inflammation and apoptosis, there is abnormal upregulation of citrullinated proteins in specific sites of body, e.g., increased concentration in joints during citrullination of antigens of the synovium in any form of inflammatory arthritis results in the production of anti-cyclic citrullinated peptide (anti-CCP) antibodies which is genetically linked. Anti-citrullinated peptide antibodies (ACPA) have been identified in the synovial fluid of patients with rheumatoid arthritis (RA). There are many subtypes of anti-CCP antibodies, but they are more important for research than of clinical arena.

These (anti-CCP) antibodies are specific for RA and are useful in identifying majority of patients with RA in collaboration with rheumatoid factor (RF) and C-reactive protein (CRP) as other inflammatory and diagnostic markers.

Data on whether there is any association between anti-CCP antibodies and arthritis among patients with psoriasis, connective tissue disorders, or immunobullous disorders are extremely limited and conflicting. Also, any correlation with other inflammatory or diagnostic markers such as RF and CRP in such patients is further complicated due to the prevalence of RA and coexistent arthritis in many such diseases.

The results of anti-CCP antibody tests are of clinical relevance only in case of symptomatic patients or if patient has a strong family history of RA. If patient has symptoms of RA and the results show:

- Positive CCP antibodies and positive RF—strong possibility of RA
- Positive CCP antibodies and negative RF—patient may be in early stages of RA
- Negative CCP antibodies and negative RF—unlikely to have RA.

Use of anti-CCP antibody test:
- Helpful in diagnosis of RA
- Additionally, anti-CCP antibody levels have prognostic significance as increased levels can denote severe joint involvement or erosive disease.

Importance in dermatology:
- In evaluation of psoriatic arthritis, to rule out rheumatoid arthritis.
- To evaluate a case of connective tissue disorder.

Hormonal Investigations

Aneet Mahendra, Ajinkya Gujrathi, Sumit Gupta, Sanjeev Gupta, Meghna Khatri, Sunita Gupta, Rohit Batra

LUTEINIZING HORMONE AND FOLLICLE-STIMULATING HORMONE (LH, FSH)

Aneet Mahendra, Ajinkya Gujrathi

INTRODUCTION

Follicle-stimulating hormone (FSH) is Gametokinetic hormone.

Luteinizing hormone (LH) is gameto releasing hormone.

Luteinizing hormone and FSH are glycoprotein hormones produced by gonadotrophs in the anterior pituitary gland. LH and FSH work together in the reproductive system.

LUTEINIZING HORMONE SECRETION

- Luteinizing hormone levels are controlled by pulsatile secretion of gonadotropin-releasing hormone (GnRH).
- In males, levels are controlled by testosterone, and in females by estrogen and progesterone.
- Testosterone can be converted into estradiol (E2) by enzyme aromatase to inhibit LH. E2 decreases pulse amplitude and responsiveness of the pituitary to GnRH from the hypothalamus.

Effect on males: LH acts upon the Leydig cells of the testis which produces testosterone.

Effect on females: LH supports theca cells in the ovaries that provide androgens and hormonal precursors for E2 production. The increase in LH production only lasts for 24–48 hours. This "LH surge" triggers ovulation, thereby not only releasing the egg from the follicle, but also initiating the conversion of the residual follicle into a corpus luteum. LH is necessary to maintain luteal function for the second half of the menstrual cycle.

Normal Range

Luteinizing hormone levels in females fluctuates. During the reproductive years, typical levels are between 1 and 20 IU/L. Physiologic high LH levels are seen during the LH surge; typically, they last 48 hours.

- *Follicular phase*: 1.68–15 IU/L
- *Ovulatory peak*: 21.9–56.6 IU/L
- *Luteal phase*: 0.61–16.3 IU/L
- *Post menopause*: 14.2–52.3 IU/L
- *In males >18 years*: 1.8–8.6 IU/L.

In child age 1–10 years:
- *Male*: 0.04–3.6 IU/L
- *Female*: 0.03–3.9 IU/L

Clinical Significance

- The detection of a surge in release of LH indicates impending ovulation.
- Luteinizing hormone can be detected daily by urinary ovulation predictor kits around the time of ovulation (1–1.5 days before ovulation).
- Luteinizing hormone level should be checked at the beginning of the cycle mostly at day 1–3.
- A conversion from a negative to a positive reading would suggest that ovulation is about to occur within 24–48 hours.

High Levels of Luteinizing Hormone

Persistently high LH levels (>40 mIU/mL) are indicative of situations (hypergonadotropic state) where the normal restricting feedback from the gonad is absent, leading to a pituitary production of both LH and FSH. While this is typical in menopause, it is abnormal in the reproductive years. If it is there, it may be a sign of:

- Premature menopause
- Gonadal dysgenesis and Turner syndrome
- Castration
- Swyer syndrome
- Polycystic ovary syndrome (PCOS)
- Certain forms of congenital adrenal hyperplasia (CAH)
- Testicular failure
- *Pregnancy*: Beta human chorionic gonadotropin (hCG) can mimic LH so tests may show elevated LH, which may be false high.

Low Levels of Luteinizing Hormone

Diminished secretion of LH (<40 mIU/mL) can result in failure of gonadal function (hypogonadism). This condition typically manifests in males as failure in production of normal numbers of sperm. In females, amenorrhea is commonly observed. Conditions with very low LH secretions include:

- Kallmann syndrome
- Hypothalamic suppression
- Hypopituitarism
- Eating disorder
- Female athlete triad
- Hyperprolactinemia
- Hypogonadism (secondary)
- *Gonadal suppression therapy*:
  - Gonadotropin-releasing hormone antagonist
  - Gonadotropin-releasing hormone agonist [inducing an initial stimulation (flare up) followed by permanent blockage of the GnRH pituitary receptor]

Detection of Ovulation

- Follicular rupture occurs 36 hours after onset of serum LH surge and 12 hours after LH peak
- Positive urine results often found only after 12 hours. So, ovulation is expected to occurs after 24 hours of LH surge

Follicle-stimulating Hormone

This helps in regulation of growth development, pubertal maturation, and reproductive system regulation both in males and females.

Effect in Males

The main role of FSH in males is to regulate spermatogenesis by stimulation of meiotic process of primary spermatocytes to form secondary spermatocytes and finally sperm formation. It stimulates Sertoli cells to form androgen binding proteins (ABPs).

Effect in Females

In females, FSH initiates follicular growth, specifically affecting granulosa cells.

Levels of FSH:
- *Normal range*:
  - Male—1.6–11.0 mIU/mL
  - Female—It varies according to phase of the cycle.
    - Follicular: 3.3–11.3 mIU/mL
    - Ovulatory: 5.2–20.4 mIU/mL
    - Luteal: 1.8–8.2 mIU/mL
    - Postmenopause: >40 mIU/mL

High Follicle-stimulating Hormone Levels

Conditions with high FSH levels (40 mIU/mL) include:
- Premature menopause also known as premature ovarian failure
- Gonadal dysgenesis and Turner syndrome
- Castration
- Swyer syndrome
- Certain forms of CAH
- Testicular failure
- Klinefelter syndrome
- Sometime in systemic lupus erythematosus (SLE) because of ovarian or testicular damage

Most of these conditions are associated with subfertility and/or infertility. Therefore, high FSH levels are an indication of subfertility and/or infertility.

Low Follicle-stimulating Hormone Levels

Diminished secretion of FSH (<5 mIU/mL) can result in failure of gonadal function (hypogonadism). This condition typically manifestes in males as failure of production of spermatozoa. In females, cessation of reproductive cycles is commonly observed. Conditions with very low FSH secretions are:
- Kallmann syndrome
- Hypothalamic suppression
- Hypopituitarism
- Hyperprolactinemia
- Gonadotropin deficiency
- *Gonadal suppression therapy*:
  - Gonadotropin-releasing hormone antagonist
  - Gonadotropin-releasing hormone agonist (downregulation)

Medical Uses

- Luteinizing hormone is available in combination with FSH in the form of menotropin and other forms of urinary gonadotropins.
- Recombinant LH is available as lutropin alfa (Luveris). All these medications have to be given parenterally.
- They are commonly used in infertility therapy to stimulate follicular development, the notable one being in IVF therapy.
- In some cases, FSH is used in ovulation induction for reversal of anovulation as well.
- Often, hCG medication is used as an LH substitute because it activates the same receptor. Medically used HCG is derived from urine of pregnant women, is less costly, and has a longer half-life than LH.

Sampling Time

In females, preferred sampling time is day 2–3 of the menstrual cycle.

Interpretation to test ovarian function:
- <10 IU/L—normal
- <15 IU/L—conception possible [diminished ovarian reserve (DOR)]
- 15–25 IU/L—conception failure rate is high
- >25 IU/L—near zero chance of pregnancy

Follicle-stimulating hormone is a better indicator for assessment of ovarian reserve because it rises early and rapidly than LH.

Cost: It is around ₹500 in India for LH/FSH, but may slightly vary from laboratory to laboratory.

PROLACTIN

Sumit Gupta, Sanjeev Gupta

- Prolactin (PRL) or luteotropic hormone or luteotropin is a protein, best known for its role in enabling mammals (and birds), usually females to produce milk.
- Prolactin is secreted from the pituitary gland in response to eating, sexual activity, estrogen therapy ovulation, and breast feeding.
- It is secreted in pulsatile form. It plays an essential role in metabolism, regulation of the immune system and pancreatic development, hematopoiesis, and angiogenesis.
- Prolactin receptors are present in mammary glands, ovaries, pituitary, heart, lung, thymus, spleen, liver, pancreas, kidney, adrenal gland, uterus, skeletal muscle, and skin areas of the central nervous system (CNS).

Prolactin: PRL known primarily as a lactogenic hormone but also has an immunomodulatory action.

- It has a role in reproduction, calcium metabolism, osmoregulation, and behavior. PRL has multiple immunostimulatory effects and promotes autoimmunity.
- It increases the synthesis of interferon (IFN)-gamma and interleukin-2 (IL-2) by T helper 1 (Th1) lymphocytes and activates Th2 lymphocytes with autoantibody production.
- Evidence for a relationship between PRL levels and disease activity exists for SLE, rheumatoid arthritis (RA), Reiter's syndrome, and psoriasis with scarce reports in the literature regarding the significance of PRL in alopecia areata and vitiligo.
- The catagen-inducing effects of PRL on human hair growth may help explain the telogen effluvium seen in patients with hyperprolactinemia.

- Prolactin has been suggested to act as an autocrine hair growth modulator with catagen promoting functions.
- Prolactin has multiple immunostimulatory effects and promotes autoimmunity.
- Prolactin increases the synthesis of IL-6 and IL-2 which are a proinflammatory cytokines, that play an important role in melanocytic cytotoxicity in vitiligo patients.

Prolactin levels (**Table 1**) may be checked as part of sex hormones dysfunction workup, as elevated PRL secretion can suppress the secretion of GnRH, FSH, and LH leading to hypogonadism.

Elevated levels of PRL leads to decrease in the levels of sex hormones—estrogen in women and testosterone in men.

Hyperprolactinemia: PRL at 25 µg/L for women and 20 µg/L for men (**Fig. 1**).

It is associated with:
- Hypoestrogenism
- Anovulatory infertility
- Oligomenorrhea

TABLE 1: Normal prolactin values.	
Proband	**Prolactin (µg/L)**
Women, follicular phase (*n* = 803)	12.1
Women, luteal phase (*n* = 699)	13.9
Women, midcycle (*n* = 53)	17
Women, whole cycle (*n* = 1,555)	13.0
Women, pregnant, first trimester (*n* = 39)	16
Women, pregnant, second trimester (*n* = 52)	49
Women, pregnant, third trimester (*n* = 54)	113
Men, 21–30 (*n* = 50)	9.2
Men, 31–40 (*n* = 50)	7.1
Men, 41–50 (*n* = 50)	7.0
Men, 51–60 (*n* = 50)	6.2
Men, 61–70 (*n* = 50)	6.9

Note: This table mostly pertains to evaluation of hyperandrogenism/anovulatory.

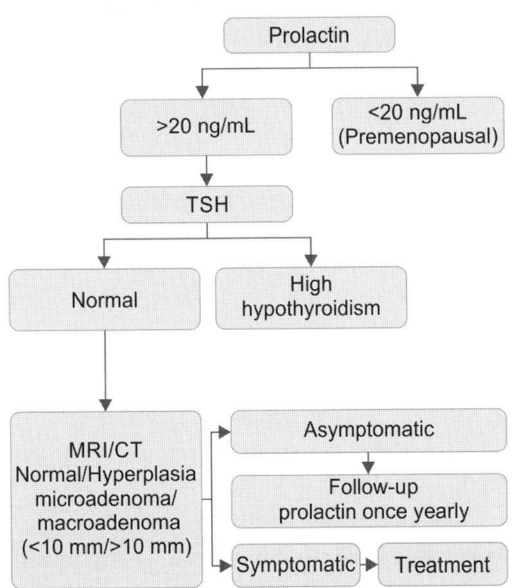

FIG. 1: Approach to a patient with hyperprolactinemia. (CT: computed tomography; MRI: magnetic resonance imaging; TSH: thyroid stimulating hormone)

- Amenorrhea
- Galactorrhea
- Loss of libido in women
- Erectile dysfunction and loss of libido in men

Clinical features of hypoprolactinemia (levels below 5 μg/L):

- *In women*: Ovarian dysfunction
- *In men*:
  - Arteriogenic erectile dysfunction
  - Premature ejaculation
  - Oligozoospermia
  - Asthenospermia
  - Hypofunction of seminal vesicles
  - Hypoandrogenism

DEHYDROEPIANDROSTERONE

Sanjeev Gupta, Meghna Khatri

Dehydroepiandrosterone (DHEA) or androstenolone is one of the most abundant endogenous steroids in humans which is produced by the zona reticularis of the

TABLE 2: Androgen production.

Androgen	Adrenal	Ovary
Androstenedione	50%	50%
Testosterone	25%	25%
DHEA	90%	10%
DHEAS	100%	–

(DHEA-S: dehydroepiandrosterone-sulfate)

adrenal cortex (90%) which is under the control of adrenocorticotropic hormone (ACTH) and by the gonads (10%) under the control of GnRH (**Table 2**).

- It is also produced by the brain (Hypothalamic astrocytes). DHEA is synthesized from cholesterol via the enzymes-cholesterol side-chain cleavage enzyme and 17α-hydroxylase.
- It functions as a metabolic intermediate in the biosynthesis of the androgen and estrogen sex steroids.
- Dehydroepiandrosterone and androstenedione, although relatively weak androgens, are responsible for the androgenic effects of adrenarche, early pubic and axillary hair growth, adult-type body odor, increased oiliness of hair and skin, and mild acne.
- Dehydroepiandrosterone is a weak estrogen transformed into potent estrogens such as E2 in certain tissues such as the vagina and thereby produces estrogenic effects.
- Approximately 50–70% of circulating DHEA originates from desulfation of DHEA-sulfate (DHEA-S) in peripheral tissues. Women with PCOS tend to have elevated levels of DHEA-S.

Normal blood levels of DHEA-S can differ by sex and age (**Table 3**).

Signs and symptoms of high levels of DHEA in women:

- Menstrual irregularities
- Infertility
- Weight gain
- Hirsutism
- Deep voice

- Excessive acne
- Baldness
- Clitoromegaly
- Reduction in breast tissue
- High levels of DHEA may not be as noticeable in men.
- High levels of DHEA-S in children can cause boys and girls to get early pubic or underarm hair.

Low level may be associated with:
- Diabetes
- Dementia
- Trouble getting or keeping an erection
- Low sex drive
- Osteoporosis
- Lupus
- Acquired immunodeficiency syndrome (AIDS)
- Chronic fatigue syndrome

An increase in DHEA-S may be due to:
- Congenital adrenal hyperplasia

TABLE 3: Typical normal ranges of DHEA-S.		
Age (years)	Levels in females (µmol/L)	Levels in males (µmol/L)
18–19	3.92–10.66	2.92–11.91
20–29	1.75–10.26	7.56–17.28
30–39	1.22–7.29	3.24–14.04
40–49	0.86–6.48	2.56–14.31
50–59	0.70–5.40	1.89–8.37
60–69	0.35–3.51	1.13–7.83
69 and older	0.46–2.43	0.76–4.72

(DHEA-S: dehydroepiandrosterone-sulfate)

- A tumor of the adrenal gland which can be benign or malignant.
- Polycystic ovary syndrome
- Body changes of a girl in puberty happening earlier than normal (**Fig. 2**).

A decrease in DHEA-S may be due to:
- Adrenal insufficiency and Addison's disease
- Hypopituitarism
- Taking glucocorticoid medicine

DEHYDROEPIANDROSTERONE-SULFATE AND SKIN

Frequent application of DHEA gel or lotion has been shown to improve collagen production which has also been seen in experimental models. In future, DHEA can act as skin antiaging agent.

It is suggested that the low DHEA and DHEA-S levels caused by long-term corticosteroid use might indicate a potential for DHEA replacement for the prevention of skin atrophy and other catabolic corticosteroid changes.

Intravaginally administered DHEA can be used to treat atrophic vaginitis and postmenopausal urogenital atrophy and sexual function.

Clinical Application

In PCOS and hirsutism: DHEA-S > 200 µg/dL

Laboratory Evaluation

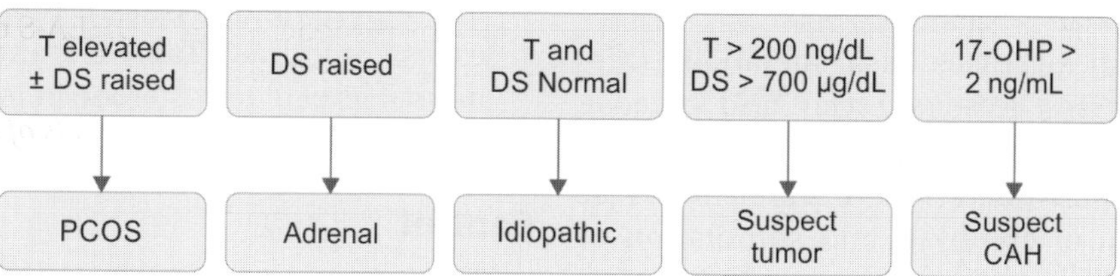

FIG. 2: Interpretation of levels of testosterone and its derivatives.
(T: testosterone; DS: dehydroepiandrosterone sulfate; CAH: congenital adrenal hyperplasia; 17-OHP: 17-hydroxyprogesterone; PCOS: polycystic ovary syndrome)

TESTOSTERONE

Sumit Gupta, Sanjeev Gupta

INTRODUCTION

- Testosterone (T) is an androgen steroid hormone found in mammals, reptiles, birds, and other vertebrates.
- In mammals, it is secreted mainly by the testes in males and the ovaries in females.
- Some amounts of testosterone are also secreted by the adrenal glands and fat cells.
- It is primarily a male hormone having anabolic effect and helps in proper functioning of reproductive system.
- Adult male testosterone level is 7–8 times higher than that of adult females.
- Females are also very sensitive to testosterone.

It is secreted from interstitial cells of Leydig between seminiferous tubules in testis and small amounts are secreted by adrenal glands in males.

HEALTH EFFECTS

- Androgens have anabolic effect which promote protein synthesis and growth of tissues with androgen receptors, e.g., bone and muscles.
- It has virilizing effect causing maturation of the sex organs, particularly the penis and the formation of the scrotum in the fetus, and after birth (usually at puberty) a deepening of the voice, and other secondary sexual characters.
- It also increases basal metabolic rate, increases glycogenolysis and glucose uptake by cells, reduces calcium and phosphate levels which leads to union of epiphysis and stimulation of erythropoiesis.

It is degraded by conjugation in liver and excreted in urine or bile salts.

PRODUCTION

- The process of production of testosterone begins in the Leydig cells in the testes which convert cholesterol into testosterone.
- Luteinizing hormone is the main hormone responsible for regulation of testosterone production.
- It is formed by its precursors—DHEA and androstenedione. Androstenedione is converted to testosterone by the enzyme 17β-hydroxysteroid dehydrogenase.
- Most of the testosterone is in bound form with sex hormone-binding globulin (SHBG) in plasma (97%), only 3% remains free.
- It is bound 65% to SHBG and 33% bound weakly to albumin. So, decrease in serum protein may cause increase in free testosterone. The small amounts of free testosterone in the blood act at the level of the tissues, primarily the seminal vesicles, bone, muscle, and prostate gland.
- At the cellular level sebaceous gland, hair follicle, prostate, etc., is converted to more active and potent form called dihydrotestosterone (DHT) by the enzyme 5-alpha-reductase (**Fig. 3**).
- Dihydrotestosterone has more strong affection to same androgen receptor than testosterone (five times).
- Some amount of weak testosterone is also secreted by adrenal gland in both men and women. These are known as DHEA and androstenedione. They have weaker affinity to testosterone receptors but can be converted to testosterone in the peripheral tissues if produced in excess amounts (**Tables 4** and **5** lists normal level of testosterone in males and females respectively).

Control

- Testosterone secretion is controlled by LH under influence of GnRH from hypothalamus.

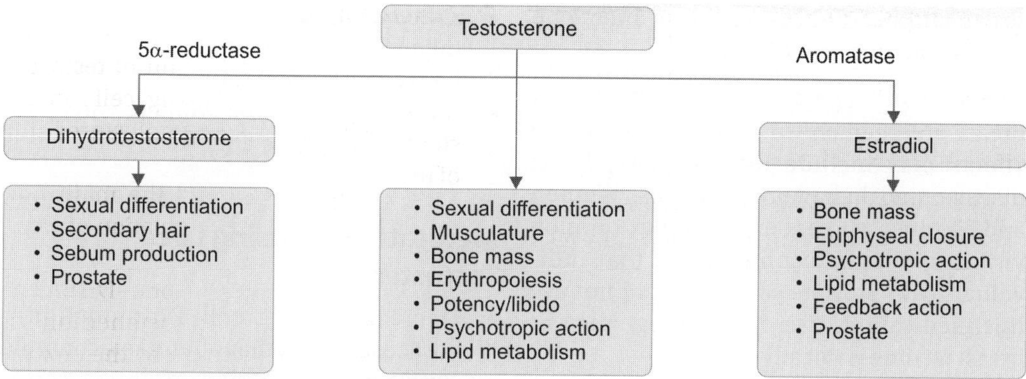

FIG. 3: Function of testosterone and its metabolites.

TABLE 4: Total testosterone levels in males.		
Age range	**Levels range**	**Mean levels**
<10 years	<30 ng/dL	5.8 ng/dL
10–14 years	<167 ng/dL	40 ng/dL
12–16 years	21–719 ng/dL	190 ng/dL
13–17 years	25–912 ng/dL	370 ng/dL
13–17 years	110–975 ng/dL	550 ng/dL
≥18 years	250–1,100 ng/dL	630 ng/dL

TABLE 5: Level in females.	
Age (years)	**Testosterone levels (ng/dL)**
17–18	20–75
19 years and older	8–60

- T has negative feedback on the hypothalamus and weaker effect on anterior pituitary.
- Other factors affecting secretion—weight loss, zinc deficiency, aging, dominance challenge, sleep, training, licorice, and antiandrogens.

Factors affecting testosterone levels may include:
- *Age*: Decreases with age referred to as andropause or late-onset hypogonadism
- *Exercise*: Resistance training increases testosterone levels

- Vitamin A and D and Zinc deficiency may lead to suboptimal plasma testosterone levels.
- *Weight loss*: It may result in an increase in testosterone levels. Fat cells synthesize the enzyme aromatase, which converts testosterone—the male sex hormone into E2—the female sex hormone. However, no clear association between body mass index and testosterone levels has been found.

MEDICAL USES OF TESTOSTERONE

Below may be off-label indications:
- Treatment of hypogonadism
- Correcting erectile dysfunction
- Correcting osteoporosis
- Encouraging penile enlargement
- Encouraging height growth
- Encouraging bone marrow stimulation and reversing the effects of anemia and appetite stimulation

Routes of administration for testosterone:
- Injectable (such as testosterone cypionate or testosterone enanthate in oil)
- Oral, buccal, transdermal skin patches, transdermal creams, and gels

A number of lawsuits are currently underway against testosterone manufacturers, alleging a significantly increased rate of stroke and heart attack in elderly men who use testosterone supplements.

Common side effects: Acne, swelling, and breast enlargement in males. Serious side effects may include liver toxicity, heart disease, and behavioral changes. Women and children who are exposed may develop virilization. It is recommended that individuals with prostate cancer should not use this medication. Use during pregnancy or breast feeding is not advised.

Recommendation for testing: A serum sample for total testosterone determination should be obtained between 0800 and 0900 hour in females a pooled sample to be taken (take three samples at half an hour gap, mix them, and send to laboratory. Preferably in cold chain).

Common alterations in SHBG affect total T levels—
- ↑ SHBG, ↑ Total T—aging, hepatitis, cirrhosis, estrogens, human immuno-deficiency virus (HIV), anticonvulsant, and hyperthyroidism.
- ↓ SHBG, ↓ Total T—anabolic steroids, acromegaly, glucocorticoids/progestins, hypothyroidism, low protein (nephrotic), and moderate obesity.

Abnormally high testosterone levels can be caused by (**Fig. 2**):
- *Tumors*: Adrenal and testicular tumors may cause abnormally high testosterone
- Anabolic steroid abuse by athletes and body builders
- *Testosterone supplementation*: As a part of testosterone replacement therapy (TRT)

Possible causes of high testosterone levels in women include:
- *Polycystic ovarian syndrome*: PCOS is a common cause of infertility in women. PCOS is also associated with obesity and insulin resistance (IR).
- Congenital adrenal hyperplasia (CAH)

- *Adrenal or ovarian cancers*: Extremely high testosterone levels >200 ng/dL may be seen in cases of cancer.
- *Anabolic steroid use*: Women who abuse steroids may have abnormally high levels of testosterone.

Medications Causing Low Testosterone

- Decrease Leydig cell T production—corticosteroids, ethanol, and ketoconazole
- Bind to the androgen receptor—spironolactone, flutamide, and cimetidine
- Decrease gonadotropin secretion—corticosteroids, ethanol, estrogens and progestins, or drugs that raise PRL (opiates, metoclopramide, and psychotherapy medication)
- Decreases conversion of testosterone to DHT-finasteride.

CLINICAL FEATURES OF TESTOSTERONE DEFICIENCY

Decreased muscle bulk/power, abdominal obesity, loss of libido, hot flushes/palpitations, decreased body hair, anemia, subfertility, subnormal genital size, loss of pubic hair, erectile dysfunction, sexual dysfunction, depression, reduced well-being, low self-esteem, poor concentration/drive, small penis, sparse pubic hair, subfertility, decrease sexual drive, osteoporosis, raised lipids, IR, and sarcopenia.

Testicular failure can be primary or secondary: Hypergonadotropic hypogonadism/primary testicular failure—It is because of testicular cause which leads to decreased production of testosterone inspite of high FSH and LH.

Secondary testicular failure/hypogonadotropic hypogonadism—It is because of failure of pituitary stimulation, leading to decrease in LH and FSH, and low testosterone.

Primary testosterone deficiency (TD) defect in testis—(1) Klinefelter syndrome, (2) XX male (sex reversal), (3) Noonan syndrome (male Turner syndrome), (4) myotonic dystrophy, (5) congenital anorchia (vanishing testis syndrome), (6) Sertoli-cell-only syndrome, (7) Acquired germinal cell aplasia, (8) Orchitis, and (9) Others—HIV, Drugs, and X-ray therapy (XRT).

Secondary TD (defect in pituitary or may be in hypothalamus):

- *Congenital*: (1) Isolated hypogonadotropic TD, (2) Kallmann syndrome, (3) LH or FSH mutations, (4) leptin or leptin receptor mutations, (5) gonadotroph receptor mutations, (6) hypopituitarism, and (7) CAH.
- *Acquired*: (1) Hyperprolactinemia, (2) GnRH analog therapy, (3) glucocorticoid therapy, (4) critical or chronic illness, (5) diabetes mellitus, (6) opiates, (7) pituitary mass lesions, (8) infiltrative diseases, (9) sellar surgery or radiation, and (10) hemochromatosis.

Contraindications of testosterone supplementation

- Untreated or suspected carcinoma of prostate [prostate specific antigen (PSA) of >4 ng/mL or PSA of 3 ng/mL in patient with high risk for prostate cancer]
- Moderate-to-severe symptoms of benign prostatic hyperplasia (BPH)
- Breast cancer
- Liver tumor
- Significant polycythemia
- Severe cardiac failure
- Untreated sleep apnea

Treatment of TD without Testosterone

- Clomiphene citrate blocks estrogen receptors in the hypothalamus and pituitary and increases GnRH, LH, and FSH release. But there is no consistent effect on seminal parameters or pregnancy rates.
- Aromatase inhibitor (AI) is used for secondary hypogonadism as alternative approach to TRT.

Investigations to be performed in patients on TRT-lipid profile, hematocrit, and PSA (men above 40 years).

FREE ANDROGEN INDEX

As we all know that free levels of testosterone are more important to decide androgen excess or deficiency, since the estimation of free testosterone is difficult, costly and not easily available. So, free androgen index is a surrogate marker of free testosterone.
It is calculated by the formula:

Free androgen index = 100 × total testosterone/SHBG

Reference range for males is 30–150, females: 1–10. Levels does not carry much importance in case of males.

CORTISOL

Sanjeev Gupta, Sunita Gupta

INTRODUCTION

Cortisol is a glucocorticoid class of steroid hormones. When used as a medication, it is known as hydrocortisone. Disturbance in control regulation can lead to disorders of cortisol excess, such as Cushing syndrome, or cortical insufficiency, and steroid insufficiency such as Addison's disease.

Total serum cortisol, 24 hour urinary free cortisol, and salivary free cortisol are the main laboratory tests implied in clinical practice.

Physiology: Cortisol is a glucocorticoid hormone secreted by the zona fasciculata of adrenal cortex. Cortisone and corticosterone are the other glucocorticoids. Corticotropin-releasing hormone (CRH) and ACTH stimulate cortical secretion. These steroid hormones act through intracellular messengers and increase the rate of transcription.

- Up to 70% of cortisol in blood is bound to cortisol-binding globulin (CBG), only 20% remain bound to albumin. The rest of amount is free which is biologically active.
- It is metabolized in liver, reduced and excreted as their glucuronides or sulfates in urine.

Cortisol levels in blood are characterized by circadian rhythm with a peak level in morning, and the declining levels are there throughout the day time. A period of low concentration around midnight and rise after the first few hours of sleep. This circadian rhythm has been demonstrated in plasma, urine, and saliva.

Functions: Steroid receptors are present in almost all tissues, e.g., nervous, immune, cardiorespiratory, reproductive, integumentary, and musculoskeletal system.

The main function of steroid is to counter internal and external stressors. Any stress leads to activation of the sympathetic and parasympathetic nervous system (SNS and PNS). This is called fight or flight response, which ultimately causes many hormonal and physiological responses leading to tachycardia, tachypnea, catabolic effect leading to more glucose production from glycogen, protein, fat, etc.

They play pivotal role in energy metabolism, maintenance of electrolyte balance and blood pressure, immune modulation and stress response, cell proliferation and differentiation, memory, and cognitive functions (**Box 1**).

Laboratory Testing Cortisol Assays

- Serum total cortisol—radioimmunoassay (RIA), liquid chromatography, HPLC, and fluorescence polarization immunoassay

| BOX 1 | Cortisol and dermatology. |

- Steroid is double-edged weapon for dermatology
- Nowadays, most of the skin diseases are either steroid responsive or because of steroid misuse
- Prolonged steroid use may cause bone and muscle weakness and cushingoid changes
- Addison's disease may cause pigmentation, it is seen mainly in cases with primary causes where failure of adrenals can lead to increased stimulation of pituitary and along with ACTH, MSH also get stimulated which results in pigmentation

(ACTH: adrenocorticotropic hormone; MSH: melanocyte stimulating hormone)

- Serum free cortisol assays—Coolen's method and ultrafiltration.
  Disadvantages are—invasive procedure and stress may lead to rise of cortisol level.
- Urine free cortisol assay—RIA, enzyme immunoassay, and liquid chromatography.
  Disadvantages are pretreatment of urine sample.
- Salivary cortisol assays—RIA, enzyme immunoassay, and liquid chromatography.
  Advantages—It is a non-invasive procedure.
  Cortisol follows a circadian rhythm and to accurately measure cortisol levels, it is best to test four times a day through saliva.

Automated immunoassays lack specificity and show significant cross-reactivity due to interactions with structural analogs of cortisol, and show differences between assays. Liquid chromatography-tandem mass spectrometry (LC-MS/MS) can improve specificity and sensitivity.

Disorders of Cortisol Production

- *Primary hypercortisolism* (Cushing's syndrome): Excessive levels of cortisol
- *Secondary hypercortisolism*: Pituitary tumor resulting in Cushing's disease and pseudo-Cushing's syndrome.

- *Primary hypocortisolism* (Addison's disease and Nelson's syndrome): Insufficient levels of cortisol—tuberculosis, tumor, and drugs
- *Secondary hypocortisolism*: Pituitary tumor, and Sheehan's syndrome
- *Factors increasing cortisol levels*: Viral infections, prolonged aerobic exercise, severe trauma or stressful events, and extreme hot and cold.

Reference ranges for blood plasma level of free cortisol—at 9 AM: 140–700 nmol/L (5-25 µg/dL) and at midnight: 80–350 nmol/L (2.9-3 µg/dL).

(Using the molecular weight of 362.460 g/mole, the conversion factor from µg/dL to nmol/L is approximately 27.6; thus, 10 µg/dL is about 276 nmol/L).

Adrenocorticotropic Hormone Stimulation Test

It is used to assess the functioning of the adrenal glands stress response by measuring the adrenal response to ACTH.

In this test, a small amount of synthetic ACTH is injected, and the amount of cortisol produced in response by the adrenals is measured.

PROCEDURE

First, cortisol and ACTH levels are drawn at baseline (time = 0). After that a synthetic ACTH or another corticotropic agent 250 µg is injected IM or IV. After that 20 mL of heparinized venous blood is collected at 30 and 60 minutes, and cortisol levels are measured.

Interpretation of Results

There is increased level of cortisol usually 18–20 µg/dL in healthy individuals, within 60 minutes on a 250 µg dose.

Addison's disease: Both the cortisol and the aldosterone levels are low, and the cortisol level may not show alteration on ACTH stimulation.

Interpretation for secondary adrenal insufficiency: This can be due to:
- Exogenous steroid therapy causes suppression of ACTH produced by pituitary.
- In case of primary causes of pituitary dysfunction—There is insufficient production of ACTH as a result of that adrenal is not stimulated leading to atrophy of adrenal glands specially if the cause persists or remain untreated. In such cases, ACTH stimulation may fail sometimes. But in cases of early phases of the development of adrenal insufficiency due to secondary causes, the adrenals may not get atrophied and can still show a normal stimulation test.

This test is used to diagnose or exclude primary and secondary adrenal insufficiency.

So, in Addison's disease, the cause may be related to adrenals, pituitary or hypothalamus. These causes are classified as primary, secondary or tertiary respectively. Addison's disease and related conditions, the interpretations of results are as below:
- *Hypothalamus (tertiary cause)*: ↓CRH, ↓ ACTH, ↓ CORTISOL, ↓ aldosterone, ↓ Na, ↓K (Na and K may be normal)— may be due to hypothalamic tumor (adenoma), autoimmune process, environmental factors, head injury, and sudden steroid withdrawal.
- *Pituitary (secondary cause)*: ↑ CRH, ↓ ACTH, ↓ CORTISOL, ↓Aldosterone, ↓ Na, ↓K (Na and K may be normal)— may be due to pituitary adenoma, autoimmune process, environmental factors, Sheehan's syndrome, head injury and surgical removal of the gland.

- *Adrenal (primary cause)*: ↑ CRH, ↑ACTH, ↓ Cortisol, ↓Aldosterone, ↓ Na, ↑ K—may be due to adrenal tumor, stress, autoimmune process, environmental factors, Addison's disease and any injury.

ANTI-MÜLLERIAN HORMONE

Sanjeev Gupta, Meghna Khatri

Anti-Müllerian hormone (AMH) is used to assess a woman's ovarian reserve or egg count.

It is produced by cells from the small follicles in a woman's ovaries and is used as a marker of oocyte quantity, produced by the granulosa cells in ovarian follicles.

- It is first made in primary follicles which advance from the primordial follicle stage. At these stages, follicles are too small to be seen by ultrasound.
- AMH production is highest in preantral and small antral stages (<4 mm diameter) of development.
- Production decreases gradually and then stops when the follicles are fully developed. Almost negligible amount of AMH is produced in follicles over 8 mm size.
- AMH levels are fairly constant and testing can be done irrespective of the day of the cycle.
- The values >1 ng/mL usually signifies a normal ovarian reserve and the values less than 1 ng/mL indicate a low or diminished ovarian reserve.

As we know that females fertility level declines as the age advances, so the same happens with AMH values. Low AMH levels in a young female in reproductive period points towards difficulty in conception in the future, so, it should be managed accordingly.

Since, AMH is produced only in small ovarian follicles, so, blood levels of AMH are a measure of the size of the pool of growing follicles in women.

TABLE 6: Interpretation of AMH values.

Interpretation	AMH blood level
High (often an indicator of PCOS)	Over 3.0 ng/mL
Normal	Over 1.0 ng/mL
Low normal range	0.7–0.9 ng/mL
Low	0.3–0.6 ng/mL
Very low	Less than 0.3 ng/mL

(AMH: anti-Müllerian hormone; PCOS: polycystic ovary syndrome)

It has been observed that size of the pool of growing follicles is heavily influenced by the size of the pool of remaining primordial follicles (microscopic follicles in "deep sleep").

- Women with many small follicles, such as those with PCOS have high AMH hormone values. Women that have few remaining follicles and those that are close to menopause have low AMH levels.

Interpretation of AMH levels: There are some inconsistencies to consider when interpreting the results from an AMH blood test. Since, the AMH test has not been in routine use for many years, the levels considered to be "normal" are not yet clarified and agreed on by the experts. Also, not all current commercial assays give equivalent results.

Low AMH means that you have a low ovarian reserve, but it does not mean that you are not able to conceive naturally. Unfortunately, there are no proven ways to increase your AMH levels, but some research has shown that vitamin D and DHEA may help increase AMH levels (**Table 6**).

Salient Points

- Anti-Müllerian hormone has been validated in various populations to diagnose PCOS.
- Its diagnostic value is after the age of 25 years.

- High AMH levels are a marker for hyperandrogenism.
- Levels of AMH help in demarcation between women with PCOS and those with PCOS morphology alone (nonclassical PCOS).
- Anti-Müllerian hormone levels are higher in women with PCOS as compared to women with normal ovaries.
- Correlates with antral follicle count, ovarian volume, and severity of PCOS.
- It has consistent age dependent levels, with high sensitivity and specificity.
- Cut off value depends on the age of the patient.
- When accurate ultrasound data is not available, AMH can be used instead of follicle count as a diagnostic criterion.
- In some cases it can replace transvaginal USG.

INSULIN RESISTANCE

Sunita Gupta, Rohit Batra

INTRODUCTION

Insulin is a peptide hormone produced by the beta cells of the pancreatic islets. It is one of the most powerful hormone in body responsible for maintaining the blood sugar levels in normal range. It also helps in the absorption of sugar from carbohydrates found in the food.

Insulin Resistance

- Insulin resistance (IR) is the condition where the cells do not respond normally to insulin and need more amount of insulin to maintain the healthy glucose levels in the body.
- In IR, the excess glucose is not utilized properly by the cell leading to elevated levels of blood glucose.

- Insulin resistance may be one of the most important prime factors behind predia-betic condition, type 2 diabetes mellitus (T2DM), and gestational diabetes.

Symptoms of Insulin Resistance

Signs and symptoms of IR include:
- A waistline over 40 inches in men and 35 inches in women
- Blood pressure readings of 130/80 or higher
- A fasting glucose level over 100 mg/dL
- A fasting triglyceride level over 150 mg/dL
- A HDL cholesterol level over under 40 mg/dL in men and 50 mg/dL in women
- Skin tags
- Patches of dark and velvety skin called acanthosis nigricans

Risk Factors and Causes of Insulin Resistance

- Obesity, especially belly fat
- Inactive lifestyle
- Diet high in carbohydrates
- Gestational diabetes
- Health conditions such as non-alcoholic fatty liver disease and PCOS
- A family history of diabetes
- Smoking
- Ethnicity—it's more likely if your ancestry is African, Latino, or Native American
- Age—it's more likely after 45 years
- Hormonal disorders such as Cushing's syndrome and acromegaly
- Medications such as steroids, antipsy-chotics, and HIV medications
- Sleep problems like sleep apnea

The skin manifestations of IR can help to diagnose the condition and its complications. Skin manifestations can include:
- Acanthosis nigricans
- Acrochordons (skin tags)

- Acne
- Hirsutism
- Androgenetic alopecia (male pattern hair loss)

Skin diseases that have commonly been associated with IR and metabolic syndrome include:

- Psoriasis
- Hidradenitis suppurativa
- Vitiligo

Insulin Test

Insulin test is done in fasting state to detect the insulin levels in the blood. It is also used to monitor the treatment of abnormal insulin levels and also to monitor IR.

Test Indications

Fasting insulin test is required for the following reasons;

- To detect the presence of an insulin producing tumor in the pancreas
- To know the cause behind low blood sugar
- To identify IR
- To determine the requirement of insulin therapy as a supplement to oral medications in T2 DM

Insulin Normal Range

Insulin normal range averages between 2.6 and 24.9 mIU/mL.

Insulin Test Interpretation

During fasting, if the blood glucose level is below 40 mg/dL along with high insulin level, high levels of proinsulin and C-peptide, indicate toward insulinoma.

Insulin levels are usually low in people suffering from type 1 diabetes mellitus (T1DM).

In the primary stage of T2DM, insulin levels are either high or normal and in the secondary stage of T2DM, insulin levels are low.

In normal healthy individuals, insulin levels are proportional to blood glucose levels (**Fig. 4**). High insulin levels can be because of:

- Type 2 diabetes mellitus
- Insulin resistance
- Cushing's syndrome, a disorder of the adrenal glands. Adrenal glands make hormones that help the body break down fat and protein.
- An insulinoma (pancreatic tumor)

Low insulin levels can be because of hyperglycemia (high blood sugar), T1DM and pancreatitis.

There are multiple methods available to assess IR, including the following:

- *Hyperinsulinemic-euglycemic glucose clamp*: It is a type of glucose clamp technique and is the gold standard for IR. It measures the amount of glucose necessary to compensate for an increased insulin level without causing hypoglycemia.

  The rate of glucose infusion during the last 30 minutes of the test determines insulin sensitivity.
- If high levels (7.5 mg/min or higher) are required, the patient is insulin-sensitive.
- Very low levels (4.0 mg/min or lower) indicate that the body is resistant to insulin action.
- Levels between 4.0 and 7.5 mg/min are not definitive, and suggest "impaired glucose tolerance (IGT)", an early sign of IR.
- Fasting insulin level is >25 mU/L or 174 pmol/L indicates IR. The same levels apply 3 hours after the last meal.
- *Homeostasis model assessment (HOMA)*: Since the clamp technique is complicated and there is a potential danger of hypoglycemia in some patients, so,

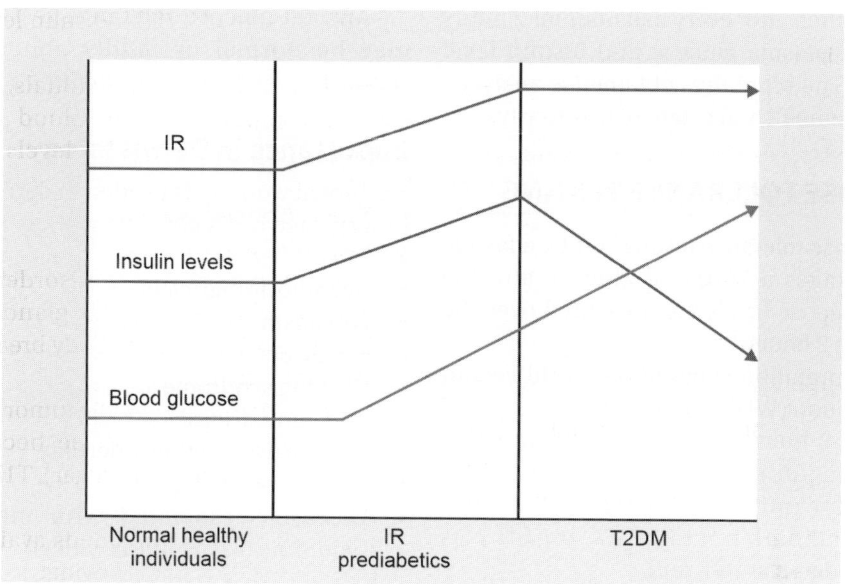

FIG. 4: Image showing relationship between blood glucose, insulin levels and insulin resistance in normal, prediabetics and diabetic individuals.
(T2DM: type 2 diabetes mellitus; IR: insulin resistance)

alternatives have been sought to simplify the measurement of IR.

The first model used was the HOMA, and a more recent method is the quantitative insulin-sensitivity check index (QUICKI). Both employ fasting insulin and glucose levels to calculate IR, and both correlate reasonably with the results of clamping studies.

- Kraft insulin patterns/protocol
- Hayashi protocol

Each of these methods have their own limitations. The lack of standardization of the insulin assay procedures prevents the comparison of results between studies; as a result, studies can be compared only qualitatively.

Homeostasis model assessment equations have been one of the tools widely used in research to estimate IR. The two equations (which use fasting blood levels) are as follows, with HOMA-IR used to assess IR and HOMA-B used to assess pancreatic beta-cell function.

- HOMA-IR = (glucose in mmol/L × insulin in mIU/mL)/22.5 or HOMA-IR = (glucose in mg/dL × insulin in mIU/mL)/405
- HOMA-B = (20 × insulin in mIU/mL)/(glucose in mmol/L − 3.5)
- *Interpretation of HOMA-IR*:
  - <1—optimal insulin sensitivity
  - >1.9—early insulin resistance
  - >2.9—significant insulin resistance

Interpretation of HOMA-B:
- *Normal*: >54.2%
- *Decreased*: ≤54.2%

How is insulin resistance diagnosed?
The testing is a 2-hour glucose tolerance test (GTT) with serum insulin levels drawn at the same time.

After an overnight fast for at least 10 hours, patient is asked to drink a beverage with high glucose content. Blood is drawn initially, then after every half hour for 2 hours to check plasma glucose and insulin level change. The score thus obtained is analyzed to determine IR and extent of its severity.

GLUCOSE TOLERANCE TESTING

For glucose tolerance testing (GTT), a fasting patient takes a 75-g oral glucose and the blood glucose levels are measured over the following 2 hours.

Interpretation is based on World Health Organization (WHO) guidelines.

- After 2 hours, a glycemia <7.8 mmol/L (140 mg/dL) is considered normal
- A glycemia of between 7.8 and 11.0 mmol/L (140–197 mg/dL) is considered as IGT, and,
- A glycemia of ≥11.1 mmol/L (200 mg/dL) is considered DM.

An oral glucose tolerance test (OGTT) may be normal or mildly abnormal in simple IR.

Importance in Dermatology

Hormonal work-up is needed in dermatology in suspected cases of:
- PCOS
- Acanthosis nigricans
- Hirsutism
- Severe acne
- Cushing syndrome
- Addison's disease
- Erectile dysfunction/infertility
- Androgenetic alopecia
- Diseases associated with metabolic syndrome like psoriasis, vitiligo.

Serum Vitamin D

Saurabh S Gupta, Rohit Batra, Anuradha Yadav

INTRODUCTION

- Vitamin D is recognized for its importance in maintaining bone health in children and adults and also for reducing risk of chronic diseases including autoimmune diseases, cancer, and cardiovascular diseases.
- The dietary vitamin D and the vitamin D formed in skin is biologically inactive. This inactive form needs further two steps of hydroxylation, first in liver and then in kidney to get converted to 1,25-dihydroxycholecalciferol [1,25(OH)$_2$D], which is biologically active form of vitamin D.

Vitamin D Synthesis in the Skin

- The effective wavelength for the synthesis of vitamin D in skin ranges from 255 to 330 nm with a maximum of about 295 nm [ultraviolet B (UVB)].
- A whole-body exposure to UVB radiation inducing light pink color of the skin (minimal erythema dose for 15–20 minutes) is able to induce the production of up to 250 µg of vitamin D (10,000 IU).
- Its precursor 7-dehydrocholesterol (derived from stratum basale and stratum spinosum of epidermis) is converted to previtamin D3.

- Cutaneously synthesized vitamin D3 enters the systemic circulation bound to vitamin D-binding protein (DBP). Serum concentrations of vitamin D3 peak in 24–48 hours following exposure to UV radiation. The distribution of vitamin D3 (which is lipid soluble) into adipose tissue prolongs its total-body half-life to approximately 2 months.
- The vitamin D formed in skin, comes in circulation and is converted into 25-hydroxyvitamin in the liver.
- This 25-hydroxyvitamin D [25(OH)D] is biologically inactive and it needs conversion into 1,25-dihydroxyvitamin D to form the active form which takes place in the kidney. This conversion requires the help of parathyroid hormones (**Flowchart 1**).
- Vitamin D helps in the regulation of calcium and phosphate level in the blood by regulation of absorption from intestine and resorption from the bones.
- Apart from calcium and phosphate regulation, vitamin D helps in regulation of cell growth, proliferation, differentiation and apoptosis. The alteration of vitamin D levels has been observed in cancer, immune dysregulation and organ dysfunction.

Dietary Sources and Supplements

There are two forms of vitamin D:
1. Ergocalciferol known as vitamin D2
2. Cholecalciferol known as vitamin D3
   - The vitamin D formed by exposure to UV light is vitamin D3. The dietary sources of vitamin D contain both vitamin D2 and D3. Thus the preparations of commercially available vitamin D though are available in both forms, D2 and D3, D2 is more common.
   - *Dietary sources*: Egg yolk, tuna fish, milk and milk products, cod liver oil, mackerel beef liver and salmon.
   - In many countries there is a policy of fortification of commonly used food products with vitamin D.

DETERMINATION OF VITAMIN D STATUS

25-hydroxyvitamin D is the only vitamin D metabolite that is used to determine whether a patient is vitamin D deficient, sufficient, or intoxicated. 25(OH)D is the major circulating form of vitamin D that has a half-life of approximately 2–3 weeks. Although $1,25(OH)D_3$ is the biologically active form of vitamin D and thus should be the ideal measure for vitamin D status but it is not, as the half-life of 1,25(OH)D is just 4–6 hours.

Normal Levels

- The preferred level for 25(OH)D is now recommended by many experts to be >30 ng/mL.
- Vitamin D deficiency is defined as a 25(OH)D levels of <20 ng/mL.
- Vitamin D insufficiency is now recognized as 25(OH)D levels of 21–29 ng/mL.

RECOMMENDED DAILY ALLOWANCE

- *Infants and children*: 10 µg (400 IU)
- *Adults*: 10–20 µg (400–800 IU)
- *Pregnancy and lactation*: 10 µg (400 IU)
  Toxicity of vitamin D can occur in hyperparathyroidism. So, vitamin D should not be consumed without advice as it may lead to toxicity.

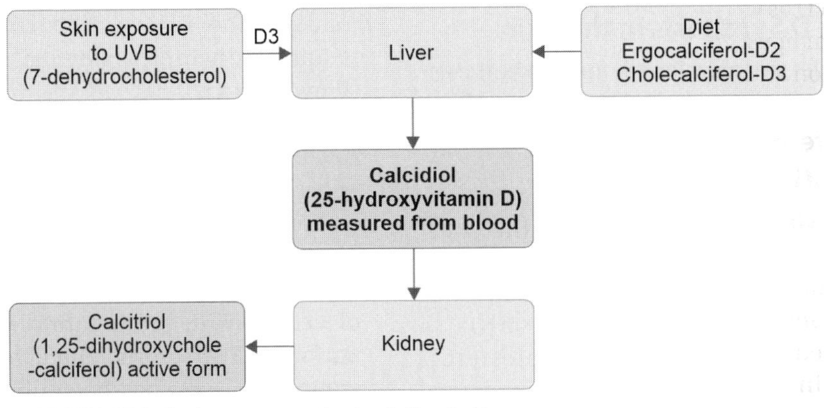

FLOWCHART 1: Endogenous synthesis of vitamin D.
(UVB: ultraviolet B)

Toxicity symptoms: Loss of appetite, nausea, vomiting, high blood pressure, kidney malfunction, and failure to thrive.

Management of Toxicity Symptoms

- Discontinue vitamin D intake.
- Decrease intake of calcium.
- For severely involved infants, orally administered aluminum hydroxide, cortisone, or sodium versenate is used.

Factors Influencing Vitamin D Levels

- Inadequate UV light exposure
- The factors influencing amount of UV light exposure on the skin such as weather, time of day, season, amount of air pollution, etc.
- Personal factors such as obesity, age, and thin skin can also influence endogenous vitamin D production. Different skin types also influence the vitamin D levels, individuals with fairer skin type produce more vitamin D as the increased amount of melanin in dark skinned individual hampers the UV light penetration.

VITAMIN D AND THE SKIN

The skin has a dual function in the formation of vitamin D as well as it also has receptors for active form of vitamin D which results in cell proliferation and differentiation.

Skin Differentiation and Proliferation

- Active vitamin D metabolite $1,25(OH)_2D$ causes increase in the expression of loricrin, involucrin, filaggrin, and transglutaminase and thus causes formation of cornified envelope.
- Vitamin D inhibits the abnormally excessive cellular proliferation and stimulates the differentiation of keratinocytes.

Cutaneous Antimicrobial Effects

- Regulates the formation of long-chain glucosylceramides which help in skin barrier function.
- Regulation of toll-like receptor and its coreceptors which in turn leads to induction of cathelicidins which help in the killing of microorganisms.

Vitamin D and Cutaneous Innate Immunity

- There are historical evidences that vitamin D from cod liver oil was used for treatment of tuberculosis as an immune-booster.
- It helps in the induction of monocyte cathelicidin expression.
- In autoimmune disorders, the vitamin D receptor (VDR) present on the antigen-presenting cells (APCs) inhibit their maturation and suppress the antigen presentation and promote tolerogenic T-cell response.

Vitamin D and Cutaneous Adaptive Immunity

- Vitamin D receptors on B and T cells have an antiproliferative role.
- Vitamin D helps in modulation of cytokine release and dysregulated antibody formation, so is of clinical importance in B and T cell-mediated disorders such as Psoriasis, autoimmune diseases like systemic lupus erythematosus (SLE).

Hair Follicle Cycling

- Vitamin D receptors are found on the mesodermal papilla cells and outer root sheath. They also have a role in photoprotection of hair.
- It has been found that vitamin D exhibits photoprotective effects in the form of

decreased deoxyribonucleic acid (DNA) damage, reduced apoptosis, increased cell survival, and decreased erythema.

Wound Healing

- 1,25-dihydroxyvitamin D_3 regulates the expression of cathelicidin (LL-37/hCAP18) an antimicrobial protein that mediates innate immunity in skin by promoting wound healing and tissue repair.

VITAMIN D AND SKIN DISEASES

Skin Cancer

- There are clinical evidences that therapeutic vitamin D has a significant protective role against many cancers and in decreasing cancer-associated mortality, e.g., tumors of gastrointestinal tract (GIT), breast, lung, urogenital system, and hematopoietic malignancies.
- Vitamin D helps in the regulation of many signaling pathways which have important role in carcinogenesis, e.g., Sonic hedgehog pathway in basal cell carcinoma (BCC).

In general, vitamin D helps in cellular arrest, suppresses angiogenesis, and triggers apoptotic pathways.

Psoriasis

- Several pathways have been established including loss of antiproliferative function of vitamin D.
- Moreover, as inflammation and angiogenesis represent cornerstones in the pathogenesis of psoriasis, the loss of the anti-inflammatory and antiangiogenic activity of vitamin D could represent another explanation to the contribution of the vitamin D deficiency in psoriasis.
- As 1α,25-dihydroxyvitamin D_3 is known to suppress the T helper type 1 (Th1) and Th17 cell proliferation as well as induce the T-regs.
- There are enough evidences that topical vitamin D therapy, e.g., calcipotriol has a significant benefit in the treatment of Psoriasis by decreasing levels of human beta-defensin-2 and 3, interleukin-8 (IL-8), IL-17F, and IL-17A in the skin.

Acne and Rosacea

- Sebaceous glands have VDR, there is an implication of Propionibacterium acnes-induced Th17 secretion in acne and rosacea, vitamin D has been shown to inhibit the inflammation induced by these markers.

Hair Loss

- Optimal levels of vitamin D delays the aging of hair.
- Vitamin D receptor promotes the ability of β-catenin promo to stimulate hair follicle differentiation and regulation of follicle hair cycle, specifically anagen initiation.

Vitiligo

- Vitamin D protects the epidermal melanin unit and restores melanocyte integrity by controlling the activation, proliferation, migration of melanocytes, and pigmentation pathways by modulating T-cell activation.
- *Antioxidant role*: Vitamin D protects the vitiliginous skin because of its antioxidant properties as it depletes the reactive

oxygen species that are produced in excess in vitiligo in epidermis.

- It reduces the apoptotic activity induced by UVB in keratinocytes and melanocytes.
- *Immunomodulatory role*: It inhibits the expression of IL-6, IL-8, and tumor necrosis factor (TNF)—leading to dendritic cell maturation, differentiation, and activation as well as inhibition of antigen presentation.

Pemphigus Vulgaris and Bullous Pemphigoid

- In some studies, related to pemphigus and pemphigoid it has been found that there is significant decrease in serum vitamin D levels in such cases.
- Vitamin D supplementation in such cases has been found helpful because of its immunomodulatory action by regulating B-cell apoptosis, differentiation of Th2 cells, and function of T-regulatory cells.

Atopic Dermatitis

Vitamin D has a role in maintaining the epidermal barrier integrity by regulating the cell differentiation, cell proliferation, and retaining the cell moisture.

Ichthyotic disorders: Vitamin D has shown its good efficacy in treating many ichthyotic disorders.

KEY POINTS

- Vitamin D acts as a double-edged sword. Deficiency leads to rickets, while excess results in metabolic bone disease. Deficiency cannot be corrected by dietary supplements; massive vitamin D dose is required.
- Normal adult level should be >30 ng/mL.
- Neither cooking nor long-term storage significantly reduce vitamin D levels in food.
- Toxicity occurs in hyperparathyroidism.
- *Toxicity symptoms*: Loss of appetite, nausea, vomiting, high blood pressure, kidney malfunction, and failure to thrive.
- 25(OH)D is the only vitamin D metabolite that is measured to determine whether a patient is vitamin D deficient, sufficient or intoxicated.

SUGGESTED READING

1. Mostafa WZ, Hegazy RA. Vitamin D and the skin: Focus on a complex relationship: a review. J Adv Res. 2015;6(6): 793-804.

Serum Immunoglobulin E

Saurabh S Gupta, Anuradha Yadav

INTRODUCTION

- Immunoglobulin E (IgE) is a type of antibody or immune protein produced by the plasma cells after exposure to a specific antigen.
- Cells like basophils and mast cells have receptors for IgE on their surface, through which IgE primes these cells during initial antigen exposure and prepares them to act when subsequent exposure to adequate amount of same allergen occurs. The binding of the IgE with their receptors activates the cells, this process is known as "cross-linking". This leads to releasing of contents such as histamine and serotonin from the cells, which produce the classical symptoms of allergic reaction such as itching, watery eyes, coughing, swelling, increased mucus production, runny nose, etc., (**Fig. 1**).
- A proper diagnostic test should be required to measure the IgE antibodies (Abs) specific to a suspected allergen in a patient rather than the total amount of IgE. But such type of testing is currently not available, so measurement of total IgE is considered to be the next best option.

The levels of IgE Abs vary constantly in blood due to various factors which are as follows:

- Exposure to the amount and type of particular antigen present in the environment.
- Current state of the immune system in an exposed person, it can be activated, suppressed or overwhelmed.
- Age—IgE production declines with age, it is maximum in children and less in case of adults.
- Number of IgE receptors on the mast cells and basophils also vary.
- Standardized laboratories with properly calibrated machines are needed for comparing data with reference levels.

A total IgE test can be done with the following symptomatic allergic reactions, especially when the potential allergen is unknown:

- Periodic or persistent itching
- Hives
- Itchy eyes
- Eczema
- Nausea, vomiting, and persistent diarrhea
- Sneezing, coughing, and congestion
- Difficulty in breathing

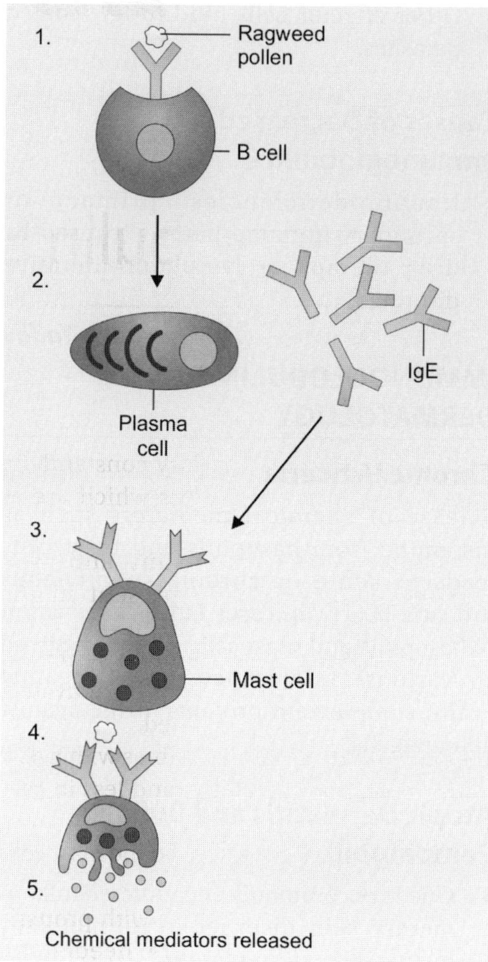

Notes:
1. The first time an allergy prone person runs across an allergen such as ragweed.
2. He or she makes large amounts of ragweed IgE antibody.
3. IgE molecules get attached to mast cells.
4. The second time person comes across the same allergen.
5. Immunoglobulin E-primed cells release granules and powerful chemical mediators, such as histamine and cytokines into the body which causes the characteristic symptoms of allergy.

FIG. 1: Steps in pathophysiology of an allergic reaction.

(IgE: immunoglobulin E)

- *Asthma symptoms*: Wheezing, breathlessness, coughing, and tightness in the chest

Sometimes, total serum IgE may be ordered as a screening test when a person has persistent diarrhea that may be due to a parasitic infection. In addition, a complete blood count (CBC) with white blood cell differential may be ordered to determine if the number of eosinophils is increased.

Testing includes:
- Testing for total IgE—the total level of IgE in the blood.
- Testing for specific IgE—the level of specific IgE against a particular allergen.

Both these can be ordered at the same time or independently.

Methods of testing:
- Radioallergosorbent test (RAST)
- Enzyme-linked immunosorbent assays (ELISAs)—now preferred
- Fluorescent enzyme immunoassays (FEIAs)
- Chemiluminescent immunoassays (CLIAs)

Normal Levels: Vary as per Age

Child:
- 0–23 months = 0–13 IU/mL.
- 2–5 years = 0–56 IU/mL (<60 IU/mL)
- 6–10 years = 0–85 IU/mL (<90 IU/mL)

Adult:
- 0–100 IU/mL (<100 IU/mL)

Radioallergosorbent test rating with specific immunoglobulin E level

Table 1 showing RAST rating and the corresponding IgE levels.

TABLE 1: Radioallergosorbent test rating with specific immunoglobulin E level.		
RAST rating	IgE level	Comments
0	<0.35	Absent or undetectable allergen-specific IgE
1	0.35–0.69	Low-level allergen-specific IgE
2	0.70–3.49	Moderate level of allergen-specific IgE
3	3.50–17.49	High level of allergen-specific IgE
4	17.50–49.99	Very high level of allergen-specific IgE
5	50.00–100.00	Ultra high level of allergen-specific IgE
6	>100.00	Extremely high level of allergen-specific IgE

(IgE: immunoglobulin E; RAST: radioallergosorbent test)

Causes of Increased Immunoglobulin E

Significant raised level will be seen in allergic diseases such as:
- Asthma
- Dermatitis
- Food allergy
- Drug allergy
- Occupational allergy
- Latex allergy
- Angioedema
- Allergic rhinitis

False high results may be seen in:
- There are reports indicating that corticosteroids increase the level of IgE.

Immune Response to Multicellular Worms

- Parasites, specifically worms cannot be ingested by phagocytes.
- Activated eosinophils bind to IgE-coated parasites via the low affinity FcεRI and release their toxic contents into the worm (**Fig. 2**).

- Other effector cells bind to IgG-coated parasites.

Causes of Decreased Immunoglobulin E

- Immunodeficiencies, primary or secondary immune paresis (caused by drug therapy or lymphoproliferative disorders).

IMMUNOGLOBULIN E AND DERMATOLOGY

Chronic Urticaria

Release of chemical mediators such as histamine from basophils and mast cells leads to acute or chronic spontaneous urticaria (CSU). In cases of CSU, activation of basophils and mast cells can be triggered by various factors such as IgG against FcεRI, complement proteins or IgE against autoantigens.

Atopic Dermatitis and Bullous Pemphigoid

- One very commonly encountered inflammatory skin disorder in dermatology outpatient department (OPD) with elevated levels of IgE is atopic dermatitis (AD).
- In cases of bullous pemphigoid (BP)—specific IgE Abs against collagen XVII can be detected in patient's serum and histopathological samples. If present, these Abs have a pathogenic role in the disorder.
- Job syndrome—also known as hyper-IgE syndrome is a rare, inherited primary immune deficiency syndrome with a clinical triad of:
  - Recurrent staphylococcal skin infections
  - Recurrent pulmonary infections
  - Atopic dermatits

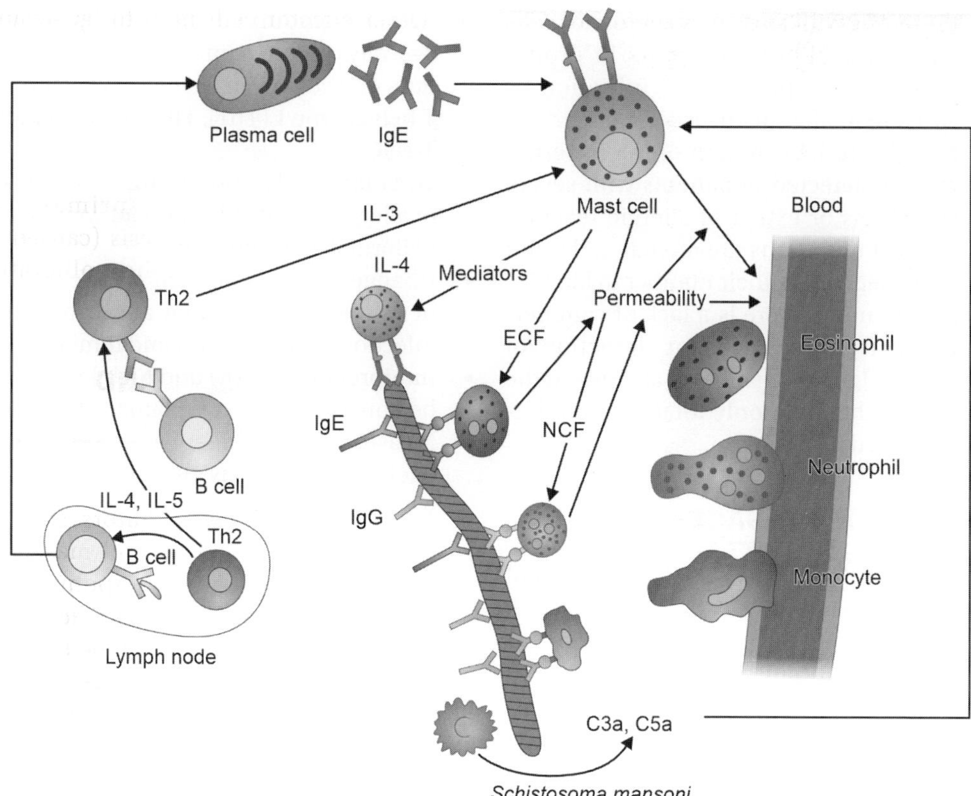

FIG. 2: Immune cascade of an allergic reaction.
(ECF: eosinophil chemotactic factor; IgE: immunoglobulin E; NCF: neutrophil chemotactic factor)

It is characterised by a defective immune response with increased levels of interferon-gamma leading to marked elevation of IgE.

How are IgE Test Results Interpreted?

Immunoglobulin E levels are most confusing and should be interpreted carefully and according to the clinical presentation. High levels may be due to parasitic infestation, allergic disorder, certain immune dysfunction, and rarely in malignancies.

The specificity of IgE is 30–95% while sensitivity is 60–95%, and it keeps varying as per age and type of allergen, and extent of exposure.

KEY POINTS

- Many a times the serum level of IgE does not correlate with the clinical findings (extent or severity) in patient on exposure to the suspected allergen.
- Test results can be misleading in some cases as false negative and false positive results can appear due to many reasons such as type of allergen, duration of exposure, age of the patient, and cross-reactivity. Similarly, normal level of IgE does not exclude the diagnosis of allergic disorder.
- A patient can have a high amount of IgE Abs in the serum but they can be clinically normal as proper binding of

these Abs with surface receptors of cells and availability of receptors in proper amount is important for initiation of cascade of allergic disorder. Similarly, a negative or low amount of IgE in serum may be detected in patients with severe symptoms or extent of allergic reaction as most of the Abs are already in bound form, decreasing their number in blood.

- Furthermore, there is a lack of commercially available tests for detection of specific IgE Abs against an allergen in the serum, therefore only total serum IgE is measured invariably.

TAKE HOME MESSAGE

- Immunoglobulin E levels are present in very low amount and contribute just 0.02% of immunoglobulins.
- Immunoglobulin E levels reach at peak level in 4-6 weeks following exposure to offending allergen.
- Immunoglobulin E half-life is of just 2–5 days, so, serum IgE can change in days or weeks from changes in balance of T helper type 1 (Th1), Th2, and regulatory T-cell.
- Total IgE levels—not useful in diagnosis of allergic diseases because of wide range of normal concentrations.
- Changes can result from a wide variety of exposures, including allergens, viral infections, medications, and tumors.
- Interpretation of low and high levels may be nonconclusive as explained above.
- Measurements of allergen-specific IgE—useful in diagnosis of allergic disease when interpreted in the context of medical history.

Anti-IgE human monoclonal Abs: They are available as commercial preparation—omalizumab. It is being used in many refractory cases of urticaria and other allergic disorders.

Serum Ferritin

Rachita Dhurat, Sunita Gupta

INTRODUCTION

The iron stored in the cells is in the form of ferritin, which is an intracellular protein. The ferritin molecules have a capacity of storing 4,000 atoms of iron. The iron molecule binds to transferrin, which is a carrier protein and transports iron wherever it is required. It should be kept in mind that both low and high levels of iron are harmful for the body and indicates an underlying problem. In some patients, it is observed that hemoglobin and serum iron levels are normal but these patients become symptomatic at the time of stress which might be due to low serum ferritin (which reflects the storage form of iron). So, these depleted stores of iron in the form of low ferritin are not able to cope up with the increasing stress, so ferritin level estimation is must in these cases and iron supplementation should be continued inspite of having normal hemoglobin and serum iron levels.

In the presence of conditions such as inflammation, infection, malignancy (hematological and solid tumors), liver or kidney disease, serum ferritin concentrations do not reflect iron stores alone and are typically higher than expected. In these conditions, it is a normal defense mechanism of the body that free iron in the blood is taken out and is transferred into the cells in its storage form i.e., ferritin. This lowering of free iron is good for arresting the growth of pathogen and decreasing the production of free radicals, thereby reducing the oxidative stress and injury. Therefore, the iron supplementation should not be done in case of active ongoing inflammation, irrespective of low serum iron. Supplementation can be done after the inflammation subsides. The diagnosis of iron deficiency anemia (IDA) in such conditions is difficult even with low iron levels. In addition, higher ferritin levels are seen with increasing body mass index (BMI) and postmenopause. In all these settings, a normal or elevated serum ferritin level does not exclude iron deficiency nor diagnose iron overload. In an individual, levels fluctuate significantly due to diurnal variation and fasting status.

Normal adult (including pregnant women) level is **30–300 µg/L**. The values below **30 µg/L** in adults and pregnant women and **<20 µg/L** in case of children is diagnostic of IDA.

Causes of Low Ferritin Levels

- Iron deficiency anemia
- Vitamin C deficiency
- Hypothyroidism
- Celiac disease

Causes of High Ferritin

Causes without Iron Overload

- Recent illness (such as acute infection)
- Alcohol intake
- Abnormal liver function, chronic liver disease, cirrhosis—check liver function tests, consider liver ultrasound scan
- Viral hepatitis—serology for hepatitis B and C
- Acute or chronic inflammatory conditions—erythrocyte sedimentation rate or C-reactive protein or both
- Metabolic syndrome (obesity, type 2 diabetes mellitus, dyslipidemia and hypertension)—check BMI, blood pressure, blood glucose and lipid profile.
- Renal failure—check renal function
- Malignancy (e.g., weight loss, anorexia)—imaging in appropriate differentials with iron overload
- Iron supplements, intravenous iron and transfusion history
- Anemia or known hematological conditions—complete blood count, blood film and hemoglobinopathy studies

- Hereditary hemochromatosis (fatigue, lethargy, arthralgia, diabetes, loss of libido, impotence, amenorrhea, right upper quadrant abdominal pain, hepatomegaly, cirrhosis, chondrocalcinosis, skin hyperpigmentation and heart failure)
- Family history of iron overload
- Porphyria cutanea tarda (cutaneous photosensitivity)
- In many clinical scenarios, serum ferritin alone might not be able to elucidate the disease process, in such cases iron profile can be useful. Changes in the iron profile in common hematologic disorders are given in **Table 1**.

Causes with Iron Overload

- Iron supplements, intravenous iron, transfusion history.
- Known hematological conditions—full blood count, blood film, hemoglobinopathy studies
- Hereditary hemochromatosis (fatigue, lethargy, arthralgia, diabetes, loss of libido, impotence, amenorrhoea, right upper quadrant abdominal pain, hepatomegaly,

TABLE 1: Interpretation of tests in iron profile.

Iron panel test	Iron panel tests					
Diseases	Serum iron	Serum ferritin	Transferrin iron saturation percentage	Total iron binding capacity (TIBC)	Transferrin	Hemoglobin
Iron deficiency	↓	↓	↓	↑	↑	↓
Vitamin B12 deficiency (pernicious anemia)	↑/N	↑/N	↑/N	↓/N	↓/N	↓
Anemia of chronic disease	↓	↑/N	↓	↓	↓	↓
Porphyria cutanea tarda (PCT)	↑	↑	↑	↓	↓	Normal
Hemochromatosis	↑	↑	↑	↓	↓	Normal
Thalassemia	↑	↑	↑	↓	↓	↓
Sideroblastic anemia	↑	↑	↑	↓	↓	↓

cirrhosis, chondrocalcinosis, skin hyperpigmentation, heart failure)
- Family history of iron overload
- Porphyria cutanea tarda (cutaneous photosensitivity)

IMPORTANT POINTS

- Estimation of ferritin levels is important in cases presenting with symptoms of anemia but with normal Hb and iron levels. The low value of serum ferritin has some clinical importance but high values can create confusion especially when there is no evidence of ongoing inflammation.
- The ferritin levels need to be correlated with iron studies and other blood indices to reach a suitable conclusion.
- The high values of ferritin are more commonly seen because of some inflammatory or noninflammatory cause rather than the actual iron overload.
- Very high levels of serum ferritin which maybe in thousands without any active inflammation can be marker for hereditary hemochromatosis, such patients can also have raised transferrin saturation (>45%).
- In some cases, excess of serum ferritin is seen without any active cause, such patients need detailed workup and regular follow-up.
- In patients with raised ferritin levels, high serum transferrin saturation denotes iron overload, whereas normal saturation levels can indicate a reactive or inflammatory cause of raised ferritin.
- In chronic liver disease, iron overload and deficiency both are seen. The iron deficiency is because of bleeding due to portal hypertension in advanced liver cirrhosis. The iron overload can be because of decreased formation of

hepcidin in the liver which works as a regulator (inhibitor) of iron absorption from gastrointestinal tract (GIT), so in cases with low hepcidin the enterocytes keep absorbing the iron despite its excess leading to iron overload.

SERUM FERRITIN AND ITS IMPORTANCE IN DERMATOLOGY

A cut-off level of 41 µg/L is significant to detect low iron stores in patients of hair fall.

Ferritin is stored in hair follicles. Low serum ferritin causes loss of hair. Hair follicle matrix cells are some of the most rapidly proliferating cells in the body. At the cellular level, ferritin levels are increased in nondividing cells, such as stem cells and terminally differentiated cells, whereas rapidly proliferating cells appear to have lower levels of ferritin and higher levels of free iron. This balance of ferritin and iron is at least partially controlled by the transcription factor *c-myc*. Also, cells enriched by ferritin show an enhanced resistance to oxidative stress, whereas cells in which ferritin is downregulated had reduced resistance to oxidative stress.

- Adequate ferritin is required to optimize the response to therapy rather than being the cause of hair loss.

Iron (Fe) supplementation should not be given in patients presenting with anemia during the phase of acute infections and flares of autoimmune disease. Iron given will be converted to ferritin as a protective mechanism to prevent the use of free iron by microbes.

- *Hemochromatosis*: Presents in skin with hyperpigmentation (slate gray or brownish bronze) in over 90% of patients.

  It is one of the earliest signs of the disease, therefore, can help in early diagnosis and intervention.

Raised serum ferritin levels (>500 ng/mL) is an important indicator of hemochromatosis.

Other skin findings include— ichthyosis like changes, partial loss of body hair (pubic region), Koilonychia etc.

- Serum ferritin is the "gold standard" for measuring the amount of iron in the body as serum iron as a diagnostic test is suboptimal. In patients with normal ferritin level CRP should always be done as both are acute phase reactants.
- Serum ferritin levels increase in presence of even subclinical inflammation, hence it is advisable to correlate with CRP. If ferritin levels are low then it is truly positive.

SUGGESTED READINGS

1. Koperdanova M, Cullis JO. Why does serum contain ferritin? BMJ. 2015;351:h3692.
2. The Royal College of Pathologists of Australasia. Interpreting Serum Ferritin. [online] Available from: https://www.rcpa.edu.au/getattachment/d2521e16-e5c3-46e8-abca-652d6838f527/Interpreting-Serum-Ferritin.aspx. [Last accessed May, 2022]

Serum Calcium

Saurabh S Gupta, Ajinkya Gujrathi

INTRODUCTION

- The mineral element in most copious amounts in human body is calcium.
- In a human adult approximately 1,200 g of calcium is there, most of which (98%) is concentrated in the skeleton in hydroxyapatite form, which is composed of phosphorus and hydroxide along with calcium forming a lattice like crystal structure.
- Rest of the calcium is located in the skeletal muscles, extracellular fluid, and in various other tissues.
- Normal serum levels of calcium ranges from 4.3 to 5.3 mEq/L or 8.50 to 10.50 mg/dL.
- Most of the calcium exists in the body in ionic forms complexed with anions like citrate or bicarbonate which is called complexed calcium. Only the ionic fraction that is free forms the physiologically active portion.
- The complexed and ionic calcium together form the diffusible fraction also known as ultrafilterable calcium as it can pass through the biologic membranes, whereas protein-bound calcium is nondiffusible.

TABLE 1: Values of serum calcium fractions.

Fraction	Milligrams/ deciliter (mg/dL)	Percentage (%)
Ionized (free ions)	4.40	44
Protein-bound	4.60	46
Complexed	1.00	10
Total	10.00	100

- Majority of the calcium (90%) which is protein-bound is associated with albumin and the rest with the globulins (**Table 1**).

Recommended daily allowance (RDA):
- Adults—500 mg/day
- Children—1,200 mg/day
- Pregnancy and lactation—1,500 mg/day.

CALCIUM HOMEOSTASIS

The calcium homeostatic system depends on several important factors:
- Parathyroid hormone (PTH), calcitonin, vitamin D, phosphate, and magnesium.
- PTH serves as a receptor arm to correct alterations in the steady-state level of serum calcium. A small fall in ionized calcium will quickly lead to a rise in PTH secretion which causes release from bone

by osteoclastic activity, reabsorption from renal tubule, and gastrointestinal tract (GIT) absorption ultimately leading to rise in calcium levels. The result of this increase in PTH is a rapid release of calcium from bone. This release requires the active form of vitamin D, 1,25-dihydroxycholecalciferol (DHCC).

- Calcitonin is secreted from thyroid gland by parafollicular cell. The action of calcitonin is reverse to PTH; it decreases serum calcium by causing osteoblastic activity and inhibiting renal reabsorption.
- Vitamin D increases the concentration of serum calcium by several mechanisms. As mentioned above, it potentiates the effect of PTH on the bone. Vitamin D also increases the intestinal absorption of calcium, as well as bone reabsorption and the tubular reabsorption of calcium.
- The serum phosphorus level also plays a role in the maintenance of a steady-state concentration of serum calcium. While there is no exact solubility product for calcium and phosphorus, a rise in serum phosphate usually leads to a fall in serum calcium.

Serum Calcium and Clinical Significance

- The importance of normal serum calcium concentration can best be appreciated by a review of the clinical manifestations of hypocalcemia and hypercalcemia.
- Hypocalcemia often leads to tetany, convulsive seizures, and cardiovascular, psychiatric, and a variety of ectodermal effects.
- Hypercalcemia is usually associated with soft tissue calcification, tubulointerstitial nephropathy, anorexia, nausea, electro-cardiographic disturbances, and a spectrum of neurologic changes from headache to coma.

Calciphylaxis is a serious, uncommon disease in which calcium accumulates in small blood vessels of the fat and skin tissues. Signs and symptoms of calciphylaxis include:
- Large purple net-like patterns on skin
- Deep, very painful lumps that ulcerate creating open sores with black-brown crust that fails to heal—typically in skin areas with high fat content, such as the stomach and thigh, although they can occur anywhere or the patient can present with nonhealing ulcers.

Causes of Hypocalcemia

- *PTH deficiency*: Genetic, acquired (e.g., surgical, irradiation, neoplastic invasion), transient (e.g., hypomagnesemia)
- *Vitamin D deficiency*: Cholecalciferol deficiency (e.g., sunlight deprivation, dietary insufficiency, gut malabsorption), 25-hydroxycholecalciferol deficiency (e.g., impaired hepatic hydroxylation, hepatobiliary disease, nephrotic syndrome, anticonvulsant therapy), 1,25-dihydroxycholecalciferol deficiency (e.g., renal failure, hyperphosphatemia)
- *Transient hypocalcemia*: Intravascular redistribution (e.g., massive transfusion with acid blood), sudden increase in net deposition in bone—metabolic, drugs, malignancy
- Increased soft tissue deposition (e.g., rhabdomyolysis, pancreatitis, hyperphosphatemia)

(PTH: parathyroid hormone)

Causes of Hypercalcemia

- Hyperparathyroidism, hyperthyroidism, bone metastasis
- Humoral hypercalcemia
- Ectopic production of PTH-like substance
- Prostaglandin-induced, vitamin A/D excess
- Milk-alkali syndrome, sarcoidosis
- Immobilization (in setting of post trauma or osteoporosis)
- Drugs like-thiazide diuretics

Continued

Continued

Childhood hypercalcemia: • Idiopathic infantile hypercalcemia • Hypothyroidism • Blue-diaper syndrome • Hypophosphatasia
Proliferative disorders: Lymphoma, sarcoma, leukemia
Miscellaneous: • Acromegaly • Familial hypocalciuric hypercalcemia • Pheochromocytoma • Tuberculosis • Rhabdomyolysis with acute renal failure

(PTH: parathyroid hormone)

Serum Calcium and Skin

- Many important skin functions like permeability and antimicrobial barrier formation, differentiation of keratinocytes, etc., are regulated by the concentration gradient of the calcium ions in the epidermal cells (within endoplasmic reticulum).
- This concentration gradient is formed by the low calcium ion levels in keratinocytes of stratum spinosum and basal layer with increased levels in stratum granulosum and again declining levels in stratum corneum.

Keratinocyte differentiation: Calcium ions (Ca^{2+}) plays an important role in keratinocyte proliferation and differentiation by regulating the transcription of genes responsible for the formation of proteins required for differentiation.

Wound healing and cell migration:
- Intracellular calcium dynamics play a role in keratinocyte migration and wound healing.
- Ca^{2+} concentration regulate cellular polarity, guidance, and migration via providing spatial and temporal information to control cellular extension and migration.

- The function of calcium in mediating cell–cell adhesion may be important in understanding the acantholysis observed in pemphigus.
- The pemphigus foliaceus antigen appears to contain a calcium-sensitive epitope, and in pemphigus vulgaris, alteration in the function of calcium-sensitive cadherins may play a role in the production of acantholysis.
- Psoriasis may have low serum calcium levels.

KEY POINTS

- Normal serum levels are 9–11 mg/dL.
- Level depends on serum protein, PTH, calcitonin, vitamin D, pH.
- Each 1 g ↓ of albumin causes 0.8 mg/dL ↓ in calcium levels.
- Serum calcium helps in coagulation.
- It also maintains cellular homeostasis.
- Hypercalcemia seen in sarcoidosis and can cause calcinosis cutis.
- Patients on steroids need calcium supplementation.
- Calcium supplementation is usually to be done in day time to prevent stone formation-crystallization in urine.

SUGGESTED READINGS

1. Elias PM, Ahn SK, Brown BE, Crumrine D, Feingold KR. Origin of the epidermal calcium gradient: regulation by barrier status and role of active vs passive mechanisms. J Invest Dermatol. 2002;119(6):1269-74.

2. Lee SE, Lee SH. Skin barrier and calcium. Ann Dermatol. 2018;30(3):265-75.

3. Menon GK, Elias PM. Ultrastructural localization of calcium in psoriatic and normal human epidermis. Arch Dermatol. 1991;127(1):57-63.

4. Menon GK, Grayson S, Elias PM. Ionic calcium reservoirs in mammalian epidermis: ultrastructural localization by ion-capture cytochemistry. J Invest Dermatol. 1985;84(6):508-12.

Serum Magnesium

Saurabh S Gupta, Ajinkya Gujrathi, Anuradha Yadav

INTRODUCTION

- Magnesium is the fourth most copious mineral element and cation in human body. It is the second most abundant intracellular cation (45% of total body magnesium).
- Major extracellular portion (about 54%) is concentrated in the skeleton and remaining 1% is located extracellularly. About 55% of extracellular magnesium is in free form, 30% is in bound form with proteins such as albumin and rest 15% form complexes with anions.
- Magnesium plays an essential role in allosteric activation of various enzyme systems as well as a cofactor for many enzymes leading to production of important substrates such as adenosine triphosphate (ATP). It also has an important role in many intracellular physiological processes such as glycolysis, protein biosynthesis, oxidative phosphorylation, cell replication nucleotide metabolism, nerve conduction, calcium channel activity, membrane stabilization, and ion transport.

The common food sources of magnesium are given in **Table 1**.

TABLE 1: Common food sources of magnesium (mg, in milligram per serving or 100 g).

Seeds	mg/serving
Hemp seeds (100 g)	700
Pumpkin seeds (100 g)	535
Flax seeds (100 g)	392
Brazil nuts (100 g)	376
Carbohydrates	
Whole wheat bread (2 slices)	46
Baked potato (3.5 ounces)	43
Rice, brown rice (1/2 cup)	42
Kidney beans (1/2 cup)	35
White rice (1/2 cup)	10
Green vegetables	
Boiled spinach (1/2 cup)	78
Avocado (cubed 1 cup)	44
Broccoli (chopped, cooked 1/2 cup)	12
Others	
Yogurt (low-fat 8 ounces)	42
Milk (8 ounces)	24–27
Farmed Atlantic Salmon (3 ounces)	26
Cooked halibut (3 ounces)	24
Roasted chicken breast (3 ounces)	22

MEASUREMENT OF LEVELS

For measurement of levels of free magnesium (complexed or nonprotein bound) heparinized plasma, serum or whole blood is used mostly.

It can be measured in urine also but not routinely done as there is precipitation of complexes of magnesium unless collected in acidified containers.

Reference level (adults)—total magnesium:
- *Less than 60 years*: 0.66–1.07 mmoL/L
- *60–90 years*: 0.66–0.99 mmoL/L
- *90 years*: 0.70–0.95 mmoL/L

Reference level (others):
- *Newborn*: 0.62–0.91 mmoL/L
- *5 months to 6 years*: 0.7–0.95 mmoL/L
- *6–12 years*: 0.7–0.86 mmoL/L
- *12–20 years*: 0.7–0.91 mmoL/L

LABORATORY TESTING

The precautions should be taken during sampling, handling, etc., which are:
- Anticoagulants such as ethylenediaminetetraacetic acid (EDTA), citrates or oxalates should be avoided as they can from complexes with free magnesium leading to wrong estimation. Similarly, zinc containing heparins can falsely increase the plasma levels of magnesium.
- Hemolysis of red blood cells (RBCs) releases intracellular magnesium in the plasma giving abnormally high values in hemolyzed samples, therefore serum or plasma samples are preferred over whole blood.
- Free calcium can interfere with the measurement of free magnesium and the samples should be analyzed as quickly as possible because metabolism can continue inside the cells for some time leading to alteration in pH which alters the distribution of magnesium.

CLINICAL SYMPTOMS AND SIGNS OF MAGNESIUM DEFICIENCY

- Magnesium depletion has been described as: "the most underdiagnosed electrolyte abnormality in current medical practice."
- Clinical signs are usually totally absent (chronic latent intracellular deficit)
- Neuromuscular signs and symptoms such as dysphagia, tremors, weakness; muscle fasciculation; Trousseau's sign can be positive (spasm in the muscles of forearm and hand after applying pressure to occlude the brachial artery with blood pressure cuff). Chvostek sign can also be elucidated (facial nerve tapping leading to facial twitching).
- *Cardiac:* Arrhythmias and electrocardiogram (ECG) changes
- *Central nervous system*: Depression, agitation, psychosis, nystagmus, and seizures

SIGNS AND SYMPTOMS OF MAGNESIUM TOXICITY

- Laxative effect, diarrhea
- Fall in blood pressure with dizziness to severe hypotension
- Muscle weakness (and depressed deep tendon reflexes)
- Severe back pain and pelvic pain
- Confusion and loss of consciousness
- From difficulty breathing to respiratory arrest
- From cardiac arrhythmias to cardiac arrest
- *Other effects*: Lethargy, confusion, and deterioration of kidney function

INDICATIONS FOR MEASUREMENT

- Suspected magnesium depletion. This can occur in the following conditions:
  - Refeeding

- Treatment of diabetic ketoacidosis
- Long term intravenous fluid replacement
- Malabsorption syndromes
- Chronic diarrhea
- Postrenal transplant
- Renal replacement treatment
- Diuretic treatment
- Hyperparathyroidism, thyrotoxicosis, and hyperaldosteronism
- Alcoholism
- Suspected magnesium excess. This can occur in:
  - Renal failure
  - Magnesium replacement treatment
  - Tumor lysis syndrome
- Free (magnesium) should be measured in patients who have low total (magnesium) and low (albumin), as they may have normal concentrations of free magnesium.

CAUSES OF ABNORMAL RESULTS

High Values

- Iatrogenic (i.e., with the use of intravenous magnesium, magnesium-containing cathartics or antacids).
- *Renal failure*: Plasma (magnesium) is regulated by urinary excretion.
- Following release from the intracellular space (i.e., tumor lysis syndrome).
- Medications that may increase serum magnesium:
  - Lithium carbonate
  - Antidepressants: Sertraline and amitriptyline
  - Potassium sparing diuretics: Amiloride and spironolactone reduce magnesium excretion

Low Values

- It can be due to decreased intake in diet (processed foods) or reduced absorption from gastrointestinal tract (GIT) which may be due to deficiency of vitamin D.
- In acute or chronic cases of diarrhea and vomiting, e.g., Celiac disease, Crohn's disease, regional enteritis, chronic laxative use, etc., there can be excessive loss of magnesium through GIT.
- Increased loss through renal excretion (approximately 30% of dietary magnesium is excreted in urine):
  - Diabetes mellitus: Increased urinary output leading to excessive urinary magnesium loss.
  - Increased alcohol intake: Leading to reduced dietary intake, GIT problems, renal dysfunction, and vitamin D deficiency.
- *Excessive sweating*: On average 10–15% of total output of magnesium may be recovered in sweat.
- Increased requirements (pregnancy and growth)
- *Older adults*: Due to lower magnesium intake, decreased absorption, increased renal excretion
- *There are two rare congenital magnesium wasting syndromes*: Bartter and Gitelman syndrome.
- *Drugs*: These can cause renal wasting of magnesium by various mechanisms.

MEDICATIONS THAT REDUCE MAGNESIUM LEVELS

- *H2 blockers*: For example, cimetidine and nizatidine
- *Proton pump inhibitors*: For example, esomeprazole, omeprazole, and pantoprazole [*Food and Drug Administration (FDA) warning*: Supplementing magnesium will not correct deficiency; you must stop the drug]
- *Antacids*: Aluminum and magnesium hydroxide and sodium bicarbonate

- *Antibiotics*: For example, amoxicillin, azithromycin, doxycycline, minocycline, levofloxacin, ciprofloxacin, cephalexin, sulfamethoxazole and trimethoprim, and tetracycline
- *Antihistamines*: For example, astemizole and terfenadine
- *Antivirals*: For example, delavirdine, lamivudine, and zidovudine.

CONFOUNDING FACTORS

- Hemolysis can erroneously suggest a high in vivo (magnesium) due to release from cells.
- A normal serum magnesium does not exclude cellular magnesium deficiency.

MAGNESIUM AND SKIN CONDITIONS

- Decreased serum levels of magnesium have been reported in children with atopic dermatitis. Mg and ceramides containing cream was found superior to creams with hydrocortisone in treating patients with mild to moderate atopic dermatitis in a double-blind study.
- Magnesium salts are reported to be beneficial for the skin barrier repair, dermal permeability, hydration, epidermal proliferation, and differentiation.
- There are multiple reports of use of magnesium chloride in the treatment of hailey hailey disease, however solo preparations of magnesium chloride are not frequently available, it is available only in combinations.

Serum Zinc

Saurabh S Gupta, Sanjeev Gupta, Udya Chauhan

INTRODUCTION

- Zinc (Zn) is an essential trace element important for a large number of structural proteins, enzymatic processes, and transcription factors.
- About 10% of human proteins binds to Zn. Therefore, Zn is associated with a wide variety of organic activities such as development, differentiation, and cell growth and plays main roles in the cell-mediated immunity, bone formation, tissue growth, brain function, growth of the fetus and child.
- Zn is a cofactor for over 1,000 enzymatic reactions and is necessary for about 2,000 transcription factors. Zn-finger proteins are necessary for deoxyribose nucleic acid (DNA) interaction, ribonucleic acid (RNA) packaging, activation of transcription, regulation of apoptosis, folding and assembly of protein, and lipid binding.

Dietary sources (mg/100 g):
- *Oysters*: 25
- *Meat*: 5.2
- *Nuts*: 3
- *Shell fish*: 2.7
- *Eggs*: 1.3
- *Milk products*: 1.2
- *Cereals*: 1
- *Fish*: 0.8
- *Green vegetables*: 0.4

Recommended dietary allowance:
- *Infants*:
  - 0–6 months: 2 mg/day
  - 7–12 months: 3 mg/day
- *Children*:
  - 1–3 years: 3 mg/day
  - 4–8 years: 5 mg/day
  - 9–13 years: 8 mg/day
- *Adolescents and adults*:
  - Males age 14 and over: 11 mg/day
  - Females age 14–18 years: 9 mg/day
  - Pregnant and lactating mothers: 25 mg/day

PHYSIOLOGICAL FUNCTIONS OF ZINC

- *Biochemical functions*: Cofactor for enzymes, activity of Zn-finger proteins
- *Cellular functions*: Growth and cell development, cell membrane integrity, tissue growth and repair, wound healing
- *Immunological functions*: Function of neutrophils, T cells, B cells, and NK cells

- *Endocrinological functions*: Spermatogenesis, pancreatic function—insulin storage and release, prolactin secretion
- *Neurological function*: Cognition, memory, taste acuity, vision
- *Hematological function*: Coagulation factors
- *Skeletal function*: Bone mineralization
- *Zn and immunity*: Deficiency causes impaired phagocytic function, lymphocyte depletion, decreased immunoglobulin production, a reduction in the T4+/T8+ ratio, and decreased interleukin (IL)-2 production.

It also play important roles in pathogenesis of some dermatological disorders. Zn can be used as effective agent for treatment of some skin and hair disorders.

An average human body contains 2–3 grams of zinc. Skin along with liver is the third most Zn-abundant tissue in the body (skeletal muscle 60%, bones 30%, liver 5%, and skin 5%). The epidermis contains more Zn as compared to the dermis. In the epidermis, Zn is mostly concentrated in the stratum spinosum. Zn concentration in the upper dermis is higher than that in the lower dermis as Zn is present in the granules of mast cells (MCs) and MCs are more abundant in the upper dermis than in the lower dermis.

Plasma Zn levels (before breakfast):
- *Normal*: 60–100 µg/dL
- *Moderate deficiency*: 40–60 µg/dL
- *Severe deficiency*: <40 µg/dL
  (In patients with mild deficiency, plasma concentration may be within the normal range)

Zinc deficiency may cause: Diarrhea, loss of appetite, delayed wound healing, unexplained weight loss, lack of alertness, decreased sense of smell and taste, erectile dysfunction, alopecia, nail dystrophy,

oligospermia, decreased sperm mobility, and decreased immunity.

TYPES OF ZINC PREPARATIONS AND ZINC CONTENT

- *Zn oxide*: Tablet size 100 mg, 80% elemental Zn (80 mg)
- *Zn acetate*: Tablet size 50 mg, 30% elemental Zn (15 mg)
- *Zn sulfate*: Tablet size 110 mg, 23% elemental Zn (25 mg)
- *Zn sulfate:* Tablet size 220 mg, 23% elemental Zn (50 mg)
- *Zn gluconate*: Tablet size 50 mg, 14.3% Zn elemental Zn (7 mg)
- *Zn gluconate*: Tablet size 100 mg, 14.3% Zn elemental Zn (14 mg)

Most of above forms are water soluble. There are many other preparations of Zn too. Out of these, Zn sulfate is the cheapest.

Zinc supplements:
- *Infants and children*: 0.5–1 mg/kg/24 h in 1–3 doses
- *Adults*: 25–50 mg/dose tid

ZINC TOXICITY

- *Acute Zn toxicity*: Gastrointestinal tract (GIT) disturbances
- *Chronic Zn toxicity*: Interferes with absorption of other essential elements such as calcium.
- *Causes of acute toxicity*: Ingestion, intravenous (IV) infusion, IV contamination during hemodialysis
- Zn chloride has caustic action and can cause lacerations and dermatitis of the exposed skin. Zn pyrithione, found in shampoos, also is reported to cause dermatitis.
- Zn chloride and Zn sulfate can cause significant eye injuries.

Specific Treatment of Zinc Toxicity

- *Dimercaprol*: 2.5–5 mg/kg deep intramuscularly (IM) every 4 hours for 2 days, then 2.5 mg/kg × 2 for 7–14 days.
- *Penicillamine*: 250 mg to 2 g daily orally in divided doses.

CONCLUSION AND ZINC THERAPY IN DERMATOLOGY

- Zn, elemental or in its various forms (salts), has been used in dermatology as a therapeutic modality since centuries.
- Topical preparations like Zn oxide, calamine, or Zn pyrithione have been in use as photoprotecting, soothing agents, or as active ingredient of antidandruff shampoos respectively.
- Its use has also expanded over the years for a number of dermatological conditions including infections as an immunomodulator (warts, leishmaniasis), inflammatory dermatoses (acne vulgaris, rosacea), pigmentary disorders (melasma), and neoplasias (basal cell carcinoma).
- The role of oral Zn is well-established in Zn deficiency syndromes including Acrodermatitis enteropathica. It is only in recent years that importance of Zn as an essential micronutrient for infant growth and development has been recognized.

*The association of Zn with some dermatological disorders is given in **Table 1**.*

The followings are some dermatological disorders in which Zn plays a role in the pathogenesis or treatment.

Dermatologic condition	Definition	Role of Zn in pathogenesis	Role of Zn in treatment
Acrodermatitis enteropathica	Rare congenital form of Zn deficiency, characterized by growth retardation, diarrhea, alopecia, and characteristic cutaneous lesions involving acral, periorificial, and anogenital areas	Zn deficiency is the main cause of this disease	Clinical manifestations are easily controlled by oral Zn supplementations. 1–2 mg/kg/day for 3 months
Seborrheic dermatitis	Chronic dermatosis affecting sebum-rich areas, characterized by flaking and pruritus with underlying inflammation and hyperproliferation	Unknown	Topical Zn preparations are effective in its treatment
Pityriasis (tinea) versicolor	Chronic superficial fungal infection involving the upper trunk, neck, and upper arm	Unknown	Topical 15% Zn sulfate solution applied once daily for 3 weeks was effective in pityriasis versicolor
Eczema and contact dermatitis	Chronic, relapsing, and itchy inflammatory skin condition	Unknown	Zn oxide paste and Zn sulfate were effective in diaper dermatitis and hand eczemas

TABLE 1: The association of the zinc with some dermatological disorders.

Continued

Continued

Dermatologic condition	Definition	Role of Zn in pathogenesis	Role of Zn in treatment
Alopecia areata	Recurrent, nonscarring hair loss	Arguable	5 mg/kg/day of oral Zn sulfate-induced significant hair growth after 6 months of therapy
Acne vulgaris	Prevalent skin disorder, characterized by a spectrum cutaneous lesions range from noninflammatory comedones	Unknown	• Topical 5% Zn sulfate was effective in mild-to-moderate acne • Oral Zn sulfate and gluconate are useful in moderate-to-severe acne
Hidradenitis suppurativa	Chronic suppurative dermatosis involving the apocrine gland-bearing areas	Unknown	Oral Zn gluconate 90 mg/day showed significant clinical improvement
Folliculitis decalvans	Neutrophilic inflammatory disease of the scalp, characterized by painful, recurrent purulent follicular exudation resulting in cicatricial alopecia	Unknown	The efficacy of oral Zn has been shown in treating this disease
Molluscum contagiosum	Self-limiting disorder caused by the molluscum contagiosum virus	Unknown	The efficacy of topical Zn has been shown in treating this disease
Viral warts	Skin and mucosal epithelial proliferations caused by different types of human papillomavirus	Unknown	• Efficacious as 5%, 10% Zn sulfate lotion, 20% Zn oxide paste, and 2% intralesional Zn sulfate injection • 10 mg/kg/day oral Zn sulfate for 2 months was an effective modality for recalcitrant warts
Recurrent herpes simplex	Painful erythema and blisters in the skin and mucous membrane around the lip and mouth, caused by herpes simplex viruses	Arguable	Zn is effective in treating this disease
Cutaneous leishmaniasis	Zoonotic disease in humans and animals, mainly caused by the two species of leishmania tropica and major	Unknown	• Clinical cure with 2% intralesional Zn sulfate was comparable to meglumine antimoniate • Oral Zn sulfate in doses of 2.5, 5, and 10 mg/kg/day for 45 days was an effective and safe treatment option

Continued

Continued

Dermatologic condition	Definition	Role of Zn in pathogenesis	Role of Zn in treatment
Leprosy	Chronic infectious disease, caused by the *Mycobacterium leprae*	A correlation between the serum Zn and the severity and the type of leprosy has been shown	Rapid clinical improvement in leprosy lesions and erythema nodosum leprosum seen on addition of oral Zn along with MDT
Necrolytic acral erythema	Introduced as early cutaneous marker of hepatitis C virus and closely associated to a group of necrolytic erythemas and metabolic syndromes	Low serum Zn levels have been reported as one of the most consistent findings	Arguable
Necrolytic migratory erythema	Rare condition associated with the high plasma levels of circulating glucagon and glucagonoma	Low serum Zn levels have been reported	Oral Zn supplementation is useful in the treatment of this disease
Uremic pruritus	One of the most common symptoms in hemodialysis patients	Decreased serum Zn has been shown	Oral Zn supplementations are effective in the treatment of this disorder
Melasma	Disorder of the skin pigmentation, characterized by symmetric hyperpigmented patches with irregular border in sun-exposed parts	Unknown	The efficacy of topical Zn preparations has been shown in treating this condition
Cutaneous ageing	Seen on exposed areas of the skin secondary to significant alterations in the structure and function of the extracellular matrix of the connective tissues	Unknown	The efficacy of topical Zn preparation has been shown in treating this condition
Skin cancers	Includes melanoma, basal carcinoma, and squamous cell carcinoma, mostly affecting sun-exposed areas	Arguable	The efficacy of topical and intralesional preparations of Zn have been shown in preventing and treating these disorders
Cutaneous wounds and ulcers	Including wound and ulcer caused by different intrinsic and extrinsic factors	Role of Zn has been shown in wound healing; in addition, an association between Zn deficiency and poor postoperative wound healing has been shown	• Topical Zn oxide pastes induced rapid healing of vascular and leprosy ulcers • No role of systemic Zn sulfate noted in leg ulcers

Continued

Continued

Dermatologic condition	Definition	Role of Zn in pathogenesis	Role of Zn in treatment
Behçet's disease	Multisystemic disease with periods of activation and remission	Arguable	Oral Zn sulfate 100 mg/day was effective in oral aphthosis and Behçet's disease
Recurrent aphthous stomatitis	The most common oral mucosal disease	Arguable	The efficacy of oral Zn supplementation has been revealed
Oral premalignant and malignant lesions	The most common neoplasms in developing countries	Serum and salivary Zn levels are reliable parameters as a diagnostic and prognostic index in case of the craniofacial tumors	Unknown
Bullous pemphigoid	Characterized by large, tense, subepidermal bullae, involving the groin, axillae, trunk, thighs, and forearms	The decreased serum level of Zn has been reported	Unknown
Sweet's syndrome	Characterized by nodular and diffuse dermal infiltrate of neutrophils along with karyorrhexis and papillary dermal edema	Unknown	Topical Zn preparation may be effective in treating this disease

(MDT: multidrug therapy; Zinc: Zn)

Radiology

*Amit Mittal, Himanshu Singla, Sanjeev Gupta,
Vivek Singh, Saurabh S Gupta, Pradhuman*

ULTRASOUND IN DERMATOLOGY

Amit Mittal, Himanshu Singla

INTRODUCTION

- Jacques and Pierre Curie, in 1881, developed the principle of ultrasonography (USG) when they discovered the iso-electric characteristics of certain crystals.
- Use of imaging in general medicine began in 1950.
- In 1979, Alexander and Miller measured normal skin thickness with pulsed ultrasound.
- 1980s and 1990s, high-resolution ultrasonography (HRUS) was used for noninvasive assessment of skin nodules and cutaneous diseases.

PRINCIPLES

- USG images are based on the properties of sound reflection which later get converted to image form. The waves reflected from a particular tissue has a peculiar wave reflection depending on tissue density, structure, vascularity, etc. Sound waves >20,000 kHz are produced by piezoelectric material.

- This difference in wave pattern of images help in diagnosing many skin, subcutaneous problems, e.g., hypoechoic subcutaneous tissue and echogenic dermal tissue, and also between hypoechoic tumors and hyperechoic stroma.
- So, all fluids like blood, bile, urine, exudates, cysts, etc., appear black-anechoic.
- Solid masses like bone, stones, tendons, diaphragm, etc., appear white-hyperechoic.

Muscles, liver, spleen, renal cortex appear gray—isoechoic.

There are many modes in USG, e.g., A (Amplitude) mode, B (Brightness) mode, C (Computer simulation) mode, M (Motion) mode, Doppler mode, etc. Modes are selected by the operator according to different sites and type of structure to be visualized.

- *A-mode*: Not routinely used except in opthalmological examination.
- *B-mode*: It is most commonly used in routine ultrasound.
- *C-mode*: Newer technology, implications in medicine is under development.
- *M-mode*: Used for visualizing structures in motion. For example Heart wall
- There are many different types of probes for USG depending on the area and the structures to be examined.

- USG measurement entails the transformation of sound waves into visual images; and B-mode scanning, the method of choice in dermatology, translates the reflected waves into "brightness" values on a gray scale, which are then viewed on a monitor.

LOW AND HIGH FREQUENCY ULTRASOUND

- There are two types of USG, low and high frequency.
- For visualization of deeper structures, low-frequency USG is used and for superficial structures like skin and subcutaneous tissue high-frequency USG is used, which is called HFUS or HRUS.
- Frequency and wavelength are inversely proportional. Higher the frequency, lower will be wavelength and vice versa.
- Smaller wavelength and high frequency waves are more easily reflected or refracted in the superficial tissues than longer wavelengths. So, are used for superficial structure, which is the mainstay of application of ultrasonography in various skin disorders.
- Low-frequency USG for deeper structures as mentioned above, frequency is inversely proportional to wavelength (λ). Higher the frequency of the sound waves emitted by the transducer, the clearer the picture, or resolution, of tissues closer to the transducer.
- Depth is inversely proportional to resolution.
- Resolution is directly proportional to frequency.

TECHNICAL CONSIDERATIONS

- First examine skin thoroughly.
- Gel has to be applied on the area to be evaluated.

- It is important to use a sensitive transducer which may fit in skin contour and avoid compression of structures.
- For hairy area, hair need to be shaved; for crusted skin, crusts need to be removed.
- Lesions should be evaluated regarding location, size, thickness and depth, morphology, content calcification or necrosis if any, vascularity, and involvement of adjacent structures.

Normal skin:
- Echogenicity of each layer is different because of keratin in epidermis, collagen in dermis and fat tissue in subcutaneous area.
- The epidermis is hyperechoic (0.06–0.6 mm) the dermis is hyperechoic (1-4 mm) band which is less shiny than epidermis; subcutaneous tissue appears as hypoechoic layer with some hyperechoic longitudinal bands representing fibrous septa, findings vary as per age. Pediatric skin is little hypoechoic as compared to adults.
- Nail bed is a Hypoechogenic structure.

INDICATIONS FOR HRUS OR HFUS

- Measurement of skin thickness, any tumor-invasion, and assessment of the borders of abnormal skin pathology specially tumors.
- In case of follow-up post treatment, e.g., postsurgery, cautery, laser treatment of hemangiomas, warts, benign and malignant tumors.
- As a treatment monitoring modality in case of scleroderma or sclerodermoid changes and sometimes in psoriasis.
- To monitor the effects of drugs on the skin-corticosteroids, etc.
- Evaluation of allergic dermatitis, nodular erythema, dermatomyositis, sarcoidosis, lymphedema of the limbs, wound healing, scars, and follow up of localized burn lesions.

- *Cosmetology*: Treatment and monitoring of exogenous cosmetic fillers in the skin.
- *Nail*: Glomus tumors, nail bed cysts, subungual exostosis.
- Cutaneous/subcutaneous cysticercosis
- Any foreign body in skin, sinus tract.
- Nerve examination in leprosy.

IMPORTANT DERMATOLOGICAL INDICATIONS AND FINDINGS (USG)

- *Skin cancer*: Evaluation and monitoring of both melanoma and nonmelanoma skin cancer (NMSC) to assess the borders, depth, and vascularity.
- *Basal cell carcinoma (BCC)*: Well-defined hypoechoic area with ill-defined contours including multiple hyper-echoic (echogenic) spots (corneal cysts, microcalcifications and clusters of apoptotic cells within the tumor mass) in dermis which may extend deep, as opposed to malignant melanoma (MM), which remains hypoechoic throughout.
- Detection of satellite lesions, excellent tool to evaluate morphology, vascularization and thickness of BCC serving as detailed perioperative tool of assessment reducing the number of incompletely excised lesions and avoiding large resection, also serves as a monitoring tool.
- *Squamous cell carcinoma (SCC)*: Seldom presents hyperechoic foci within the tumor. Because of aggressive behaviour, is more likely to invade soft tissues, cartilage and adjacent bone.
- Color Doppler may show a mixed pattern with internal and peripheral vascularization.
- SCC usually have hyperkeratosis and associated with higher inflammatory process, as a result of that it is overestimated by USG.

Melanoma:
- HFUS is used to establish the tumor thickness, margins and vascularization.
- Despite nevic lesions presenting irregular echogenicity and melanoma showing homogeneous echotexture, these lesions cannot be differentiated by HFUS, which may overestimate tumor size in lesions with nevus—melanoma association.
- *Color Doppler in melanoma*: Vascularization is more intense than in benign lesions, predominating arterial vessels with low flow.
- Detection of intralesional blood vessels may sometime differentiate melanoma and nonmelanoma tumors.
- Regional lymphatic spread can be seen.

Inflammatory and infectious diseases:
- *HRUS up to 50 MHz*: Inflammatory diseases including scleroderma, morphea, lichen sclerosus et atrophicus (LSA), and hidradenitis suppurativa
- To study site, size, extent, depth, vascularity, lymph node involvement etc.
- Lipomas and subcutaneous fat may show same echogenecity but because of the additional morphologic features present in lipomas, fibrolipomas, angiolipomas may show altered echogenicity.

Morphea:
- Doppler USG has shown great promise in evaluation of scleroderma. It has been used to diagnose scleroderma by analyzing structural changes in tissue and vascularity.
- Doppler USG may further prove useful in monitoring disease activity.
- *Monitoring of treatment*: Inflammatory lesions are hypoechoic while sclerotic are hyperechoic.
- By HFUS, detection of subclinical lesions may be possible. And also for assessment of treatment response.

Cutaneous neurofibromas shows well-defined, hypoechoic epidermal lesion, just above the dermis.

Benign nevus seen as black, slightly elevated, plaque like pigmentary lesions. HRUS shows hypoechoic, homogeneous, oval, intradermal lesion with well-defined borders.

Pilonidal cyst: In intergluteal region presenting as an abscess. HRUS shows long, irregular hypoechoic tract in the dermis and subcutaneous tissue, with linear internal foci corresponding to hair fragments.

Psoriasis:
- The HFUS and color Doppler imaging: To assess disease activity and therapeutic response by evaluating thickness of the lesion and extent.
- Familiarity with normal variation of skin thickness at various anatomical sites is important.
- Color Doppler may detect extent of dermal vasodilation and tortuosity.
- Nail changes can also be studied.

Infectious diseases:
- Detection of retained foreign bodies, abscesses and cellulitis in early stage by detecting edema in the subcutaneous tissue, which is reflected as a diffuse increase in the echogenicity.
- In early diagnosis of necrotizing fasciitis, subcutaneous emphysema and deep fascial thickening secondary to fluid collections and gas in the deep fascial plane.

Polycystic ovarian disease (PCOD):
- ≥12 follicles within the ovary with a diameter of 2–9 mm and/or
- Ovarian volume ≥ 10 cm^3
- Such USG finding in single gonad is sufficient to diagnose or define polycystic ovaries.

Ultrasonography for peripheral nerves in leprosy:
- USG is noninvasive, amenable tool to study any structural changes in nerve sites, e.g., enlargement, nodularity, cyst, abscess. It can be an alternative to biopsy and much economical to magnetic resonance imaging (MRI).
- Moreover, with USG the nerve can be probed for a longer length than MRI examination which is limited to defined segments.

Vascular malformations: To know: site, depth, type—arterial or venous, rate of flow, feeding vessel and response to treatment.

Infantile hemangioma: Well-defined hypo/hyperechoic lesion in subcutaneous plane with increased flow. Flow may be high or low depending on phase.

Arteriovenous (AV) malformation: Enlarged feeding arteries, dilated veins with high flow. Arterialized draining veins with a biphasic pattern.

Venous malformation: Ill-defined lesion with mixed echogenicity with dilated veins with slow monophasic venous flow.

Lymphatic malformation: Monocystic lesion with variable size, variable vascular components. Microcystic variety present as hyperechoic mass.

LIMITATIONS OF USG

It is an evolving branch and many things need to be standardized. There are lots of anatomical and subjective variations.
- Cannot detect lesions that are epidermal only or that measure <0.1 mm in depth.
- USG may overestimate the tumor thickness compared to the actual histological thickness in lesions with inflammatory peritumoral infiltration like

melanomas and BCC, and similarly underestimate the thickness in ulcerated lesions.
- Hyperkeratotic SCCs may not be well visualized on HFUS.

FUTURE OF USG

- HFUS probes and newer techniques like spatial and tissue harmonic imaging, three-dimensional (3D) views, panoramic views, etc. may provide a much better imaging quality for better assessment of cutaneous lesions.
- The sensitivity of Doppler examination can be increased by contrast-enhanced USG, which is under development.
- Ultrasound elastography can be used for evaluation of stiffness or strain images of soft tissue in malignant tumors and benign lesions, lymphedema, and to study aging changes also. It may lead to avoidance of biopsy in some cases in future.

DOPPLER ULTRASOUND

Sanjeev Gupta, Amit Mittal

INTRODUCTION

- It is a type of ultrasonography based on the principle of Doppler effect, which is generated by imaging of the movement of different body fluids and tissues and their change in relative velocity as compared to USG probe.
- By calculating the change in frequency shift of a particular tissue fluid, e.g., flow in blood vessel or a jet type of flow over a cardiac valve, we can determine and visualize speed and direction. Color Doppler or color flow Doppler is the representation of the velocity by different color scale.
- Color Doppler images are generally combined with grayscale (B-mode) images to display duplex USG images, allowing for simultaneous visualization of the anatomy of the area.
- If the sound source moves toward the listener, the sound is perceived to have a higher frequency/pitch, and a lower frequency as it moves away from the listener.

Doppler effect: It is the change in frequency of sound due to the relative motion of the source and receiver.
- Doppler shift (Δf) = Reflected frequency – Transmitted frequency
- Doppler angle (θ) = Angle between the direction of source – Direction of sound

Doppler USG monitor tissues in motion, i.e., blood flow. Doppler USG is based on the principle that the transducer and the reflector of the sound wave are moving with respect to each other.

CLASSIFICATIONS OF DOPPLER ULTRASONOGRAPHY

- *Types*: Continuous wave Doppler, color Doppler, pulse wave Doppler, duplex Doppler
- *Outputs/Imaging modes*: Color Doppler, power Doppler, spectral Doppler.
- *Modes*: Duplex mode, triplex mode
- *Functions*: Transcranial, tissue Doppler, others.
- Pulsed wave Doppler determine the depth of the moving objects with accurate localization of origin.
- Continuous wave Doppler monitors moving objects but is unable to localize the origin.

Duplex ultrasonography is a conglomeration of B-wave imaging and pulsed wave Doppler, creating a picture of flow. It combines two-dimensional (2D) B-mode imaging and a Doppler type (e.g., color Doppler). The duplex system allows estimation of the flow velocity directly from the Doppler shift frequency.

This may be color coded (color Doppler) to assess directionality of flow, or amplitude coded (power Doppler) to demonstrate the volume of blood. Some laboratories use red to indicate flow toward the transducer and blue away from the transducer.

Doppler study determines the amount of vascular stenosis (narrowing) or occlusion (complete blockage) within an artery, it assists in ruling out aneurysmal disease, and it is the main aid to rule out thrombotic events.

Duplex is an inexpensive, noninvasive way to determine pathology. It can be used for:

- Carotid ultrasonography
- Ultrasonography of deep venous thrombosis
- Ultrasonography of chronic venous insufficiency of the legs
  Color Doppler-Colors are assigned depending on:
- *Direction*: Motion toward (positive Doppler shift) or (velocity mode) away (negative Doppler shift) from the transducer.
- *Flow* (variance mode): Laminar or turbulent flow
  - Laminar flow normally exists at the center of large smooth vessels.
  - Turbulent flow occurs when the vessel is disrupted by plaque and stenosis.
- *Velocity magnitude*: Mapped to the color intensity.

Triplex mode combines three methods: B-mode (grayscale), Color Doppler, and Spectral Doppler.

KEY POINTS

- Doppler study is used to see details of any fluid, blood, etc., like its flow, extent of flow, velocity, arterial or venous, details of vessels anatomy (stenosis, aneurysm, leaking, shunt, etc.), especially in case of Vascular malformations.
- There are different scanning modes in Doppler.
- For a good Doppler, probe should be of good quality with a minimal angle (below 60, not above 90).
- There are many Doppler probes depending on type of tissue and site.

PENILE ULTRASONOGRAPHY/ DOPPLER

Sanjeev Gupta, Vivek Singh

INTRODUCTION

Penile Doppler ultrasonography is a high-performing, noninvasive, or minimally-invasive imaging modality which helps in evaluation of penile architecture—soft tissue and vasculature. It is the investigation of choice for the evaluation of erectile dysfunction (ED), Peyronie's disease etc.

- *B-mode ultrasound*: Linear array of transducers simultaneously scans a plane—2D image.
- Doppler sonography
- Power Doppler for calculation of speed.
- Color Doppler for direction.
  A routine USG can detect any anatomical variation in penile shaft, e.g., any tumor, cyst, Peyronie's disease, etc., for vascular problem, we need Doppler USG.

ERECTILE DYSFUNCTION

- Erectile dysfunction can be due to many causes mainly psychogenic. Other causes can also be there like neurogenic, hormonal, drug induced. Psychogenic cause can further aggravate the organic causes (mixed ED).

- The main cause of organic ED is vascular component, vascular cause can further be classified as arterial and venous (known as arteriogenic and Venogenic ED).
- In the different phases of penile tumescence/erection, first there is arterial influx into the corpora cavernosa and later there is a veno-occlusion to prevent the blood from draining out to maintain the erection. So among the vascular cause there can be insufficient filling of cavernosa because of arterial pathologies or there can be early leakage of blood because of venous valvular insufficiency. So, Doppler helps in diagnosing and differentiating these causes.
- *In the arterial evaluation estimation of peak systolic velocity (PSV)*: PSV is the most accurate parameter. PSV < 25–30 cm/s, suggestive of arterial insufficiency, with 92% accuracy.
- *End-diastolic velocity (EDV)*: EDV > 5 cm/s (during all phases of erection), suggestive of venous leak or veno-occlusive ED.
- *Limitation*: The diagnosis of mixed ED cannot be made using Doppler ultrasonography because venous competence cannot be assessed in a patient with arterial insufficiency.

Indications for Color Doppler sonography in ED:
- Already excluded endocrine and neurological etiology.
- Failed trial of phosphodiesterase type-5 (PDE-5) inhibitors.
- *History suggestive of*: (1) AV fistula, (2) veno-occlusive dysfunction, and (3) Peyronie's disease

For an effective penile Doppler ultrasound, we need papaverine or prostaglandin injection in penile shaft. One should be expert in giving injection. Overdose or wrong technique may cause complication especially priapism, and one should be competent to treat priapism if it happens.

Priapism is a medical emergency, which is the persistent tumescence of penis which is unrelated to sexual stimulation, the cause of priapism can be either arterial or venous. Venous cause is more common than arterial, which can be due to decreased or absent venous drainage. Arterial causes are less common and can be due to increased arterial inflow which maybe because of fistula or tumor and sometimes metastasis.

Peyronie's disease is another important indication where penile Doppler is diagnostic. In this disease, there is fibrosis or sometimes a palpable nodule is formed in the corpora cavernosa which leads to painful erection, progressive curvature, and sometimes shortening of the penile shaft.

The Doppler study helps in the visualization of the fibrous plaque which maybe with or without calcification, fibrous plaque is better visualized if associated with calcification.

KEY POINTS

- Penile color Doppler USG is not for every patient with suspected Vasculogenic ED.
- Normal values are still not finalized.
- PSV and EDV still carry importance and may replace penile cavernosometry/cavernosography and arteriography in some circumstances.
- One should be quite competent in giving and treating complication of prostaglandin or papaverine injection for Doppler study.

CT SCAN

Saurabh S Gupta, Amit Mittal

INTRODUCTION

Computed tomography (CT) is based on X-rays. X-rays are produced by the high energy electrons released from a heated cathode. These X-rays are passed through the target tissues and then detected on the other side to obtain images.

Amount of X-rays absorbed is directly proportional to density of the tissue. So in case of bones, most of the X-rays are absorbed so they appear white, alternatively air does not absorb X-rays leading to black color.

In comparison to plain X-ray film, CT is highly sensitive as it can detect minute differences in the density making the visualization of structures better.

In spiral CT which is a new technology, consists of multiple rotating detectors around the patient with a single source of radiation and the 3D information obtained can be sliced in very thin sections in different planes.

There are various phases of CT scan specially when contrast is used.

When we inject contrast in vein, it reaches heart within few seconds, and after that it enters the arterial system, which is called arterial phase. And after filling arteries the contrast is taken back through veins, which is called venous phase.

- *Phases* of a scan refer to when the images are taken, relative to time of contrast administration.
- The chest is usually scanned in the arterial phase.
- The abdomen is scanned in portal venous phase.
- Liver lesions are scanned with triple phase scan.

Artefacts if present can cause misinterpretation. For example:
- Metal pieces seen as radiating bright streaks, e.g., sternotomy wires, aneurysm clips, and dental fillings.
- *High concentration of intravenous (IV) contrast media*: Causes perivenous artifacts around arm veins.

- *Motion*: Minimized by asking patient to hold their breath.

Tissue density is measured in Hounsfield units (HU).

$$Air = -1,000\ HU;\ Water = 0\ HU$$

According to density, some idea about composition of lesion can be obtained, e.g., whether the lesion is of fluid or soft tissue density.

Density of tissues on CT: Tissue density is different in different tissues and varies accordingly.

Air < Fat < Fluid < Soft tissue < Bone < Metal
- Air = –1,000 HU
- Lung = –500 HU (mixture of air and soft tissue)
- Fat = –50 HU (slightly less dense than simple fluid)
- Water = 0 HU
- Soft tissue (and blood) = +50 HU (slightly more dense than simple fluid)
- Bone = +1,000 HU

CONTRAST

Iodine-based IV contrast medium is mainly used for most CTs.

Conditions where contrast to be avoided:
- CT kidneys, ureters, and bladder scan (KUBs) (looking for renal stones)
- CT head (unless a mass lesion is suspected).
- Poor renal function [estimated glomerular filtration rate (eGFR) < 30]: Noncontrast CT or alternative modalities (e.g., MRI) used.

Risks of IV contrast administration:
- *Contrast-induced nephropathy*: Creatinine may rise by 25% from baseline

within 3 days. It is usually self-limiting but sometimes can complicate preexisting renal disease.
- Anaphylaxis usually occurs immediately or within 0.5–1 hour.
- Delayed allergic response may occur up to a week.

CONTRAINDICATIONS

As such there are no absolute contraindications to CT, but the main concern is of IV contrast.
- Patients with eGFR <60 but >30 can have contrast, if they are given prehydration (oral and IV fluids).
- In pregnant women and children CT should be avoided but can be done with explanation of risk and if highly indicated.

MAGNETIC RESONANCE IMAGING

Pradhuman, Saurabh S Gupta, Amit Mittal

PHYSICS

The Magnetic resonance imaging or MRI generates pulses of radiofrequency (RF) energy and an extremely strong magnetic field causing alignment of hydrogen nuclei in various tissues and body water and other fluids. The subsequent loss of alignment with time produces the MRI signal.

There are two main MRI sequences:
1. *T1: Water* is *dark*—better for visualizing *anatomy* (soft tissue structures) (**Fig. 1**).
2. *T2: Water* is *bright*—better for visualizing *pathology* (inflammation, edema) (**Fig. 2**).

Other commonly used types are:
- *Diffusion weighted imaging (DWI)*: Diffusion restriction is bright.
  - Useful for *ischemic strokes*, abscesses, aggressive tumors.
- *Fluid attenuated inversion recovery (FLAIR)*: Like T2, but water is dark.
  - Useful for *multiple sclerosis* (periventricular lesions).

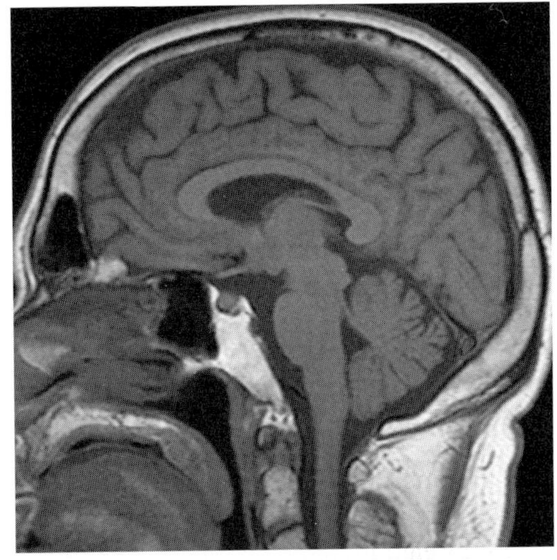

FIG. 1: T1 MRI.

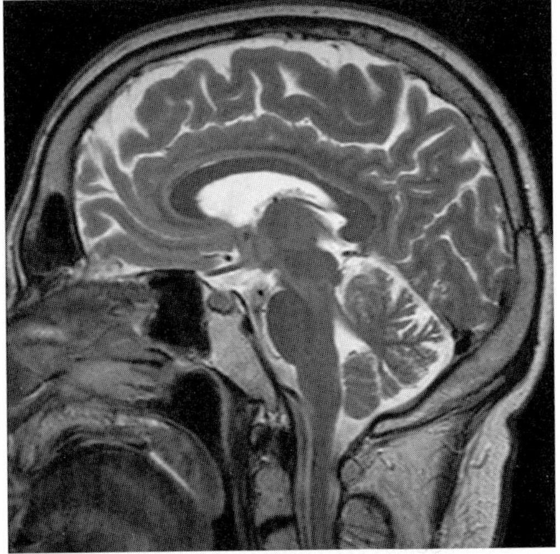

FIG. 2: T2 MRI.

- *Short tau inversion recovery (STIR)*: Like T2, but fat is dark.
  - Useful for edema in tissues, joints, perianal abscesses.
- *Magnetic resonance angiography (MRA)*: Vessels are bright.
  - Useful for *arteriovenous malformations (AVMs), aneurysms* (can be done with or without contrast).

CONTRAST

- *Gadolinium* is a *metal-based contrast* given IV.
- It can rarely cause nephrogenic systemic fibrosis (similar to scleroderma) in patients with renal failure.
- To be avoided in patients with eGFR < 30.

CONTRAINDICATIONS

Precautions/checklist to be taken care of before starting the machine.

- All foreign metallic and magnetic bodies should be removed as they can cause serious damage in case they move during the scan. A thorough screening of patient and attendant should be done before scanning. If patient is unconscious, its better to confirm absence of metallic bodies with an X-ray.
- Most of modern implants, e.g., pacemakers, cardiac stents, joint prosthesis are MRI safe, but still they must be rechecked to ensure compatibility. They cause a black void artefact on imaging.
- Patients who are claustrophobic or are irritable and cannot lie calmly and still, MRI scanning is difficult in such cases as machines generate loud noises which patients are not able to tolerate.
- Sometimes, monitoring leads can heat up excessively during the scan and may cause burn.
- Strict precaution should be taken that no one else should enter the room without proper screening. As loose ferromagnetic objects can turn into deadly projectiles if brought in the room.

KEY POINTS

- Plain radiographs are part of basic investigations and are most widely used as diagnostic imaging tool.
- They help in bone tumor characterization as well as some chest and abdominal pathology.
- USG is a cost-effective screening and diagnostic tool for evaluation of intra-abdominal organs.
- USG should be preferred in the pediatric population to avoid radiation exposure.
- CT scans are preferred for initial diagnosis of internal malignancies and monitoring of disease progression.
- Contrast imaging is now made possible in patients having compromised renal function, because of advent of non-ionic iodinated water-soluble IV contrast.
- MRI is superior to other modalities, specifically for soft tissue and intracranial evaluation.
- CT scan along with positron emission tomography (PET) scans are performed simultaneously to aid in the diagnosis of metastatic disease and help in monitoring. If PET scan is positive, we need to evaluate for false positive uptake which can create confusion. But if comes negative, it rules out presence of metastasis.
- For head and scalp midline lesions, sometimes CT/MRI are used to evaluate bony abnormalities if any and possibility of central nervous system (CNS) communications.
- In infants of 3–5 months age with the midline spinal lesions, USG can provide good guide of the spinal cord and canal as

the vertebrae have not yet ossified at that age.

- In patients of above 3–5 months age with midline spinal lesions pathology, MRI is preferred.
- Imaging modalities such as CT and MRI are also used for work up/screening of internal malignancy specially in patients with paraneoplastic conditions, such as acrokeratosis paraneoplastica (Bazex syndrome), dermatomyositis, erythema gyratum repens, and paraneoplastic pemphigus.

SUGGESTED READINGS

1. Bhat V, Salins PC, Bhat V. Imaging spectrum of hemangioma and vascular malformations of the head and neck in children and adolescents. J Clin Imaging Sci. 2014;4:31.
2. Jain S, Visser LH, Praveen TLN, Rao PN, Surekha T, Ellanti R, et al. High-resolution sonography: a new technique to detect nerve damage in leprosy. PLoS Negl Trop Dis. 2009;3(8):e498.
3. Jung DC, Park SY, Lee JY. Penile Doppler ultrasonography revisited. Ultrasonography. 2018;37(1):16-24.
4. Kleinerman R, Whang TB, Bard RL, Marmur ES. Ultrasound in dermatology: principles and applications. J Am Acad Dermatol. 2012;67(3):478-87.

INDEX

Page numbers followed by *b* refer to box, *f* refer to figure, *fc* refer to flowchart, and *t* refer to table.